A WEIGHT OFF YOUR MIND
How to stop worrying about your body size

SUE DYSON was brought up on Merseyside, and qualified as a translator before becoming a secretary. A graduate in French and English, she passed the Private and Executive Secretary's Diploma exams with the highest marks ever awarded. She has taught secretarial students as a part-time lecturer at Scarborough Technical College. She is also the author, with Stephen Hoare, of *How to be a Successful Secretary* and *Changing Course: How to take charge of your career* (both Sheldon 1990).

D1646265

For a complete list of titles in the **Overcoming Common Problems**
Series write to:

Sheldon Press,
SPCK, Marylebone Road, London NW1 4DU

Overcoming Common Problems

A WEIGHT OFF YOUR MIND

How to stop worrying about your body size

Sue Dyson

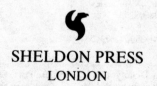

SHELDON PRESS
LONDON

First published in Great Britain in 1991
Sheldon Press, SPCK, Marylebone Road, London NW1 4DU

British Library Cataloguing in Publication Data
Dyson, Sue
A weight off your mind: how to stop worrying
about your body size
1. Women. Obesity. Psychological aspects
I. Title   II. Series
616.3980082

ISBN 0–85969–623–5

Photoset by Deltatype Ltd, Ellesmere Port, Cheshire
Printed in Great Britain by Biddles Ltd, Guildford and Kings Lynn

Introduction

This book is about living happily with your body, whatever its shape or size. It isn't a diet book; nor is it another attempt to promote the old 'fat is fantastic' doctrine which many people find so difficult to accept.

Fat *isn't* fantastic. In fact, it is neither good nor bad. Fat is simply fat. In an ideal world, your dress size would be of no more consequence than your shoe size.

But this isn't an ideal world, and large people everywhere know the anguish of being made to feel different, and somehow imperfect. Being quite large myself, and very stubborn besides, I am just not prepared to accept the common implication that being large and being inferior are one and the same thing. It is all nonsense – like saying that blue eyes are better than brown ones, or blondes are worth more than redheads. The size of a person's body has nothing to do with the personality and the intellect inside.

More and more people are asserting their right to be big and happy – denying that there should be any relationship between body size and the quality of an individual's life. Organizations like the London Fat Women's Group are forming to bring the issues out into the open, forcing ordinary people to rethink their prejudices and giving fat people the confidence to walk tall in a world where thin has meant successful for so long.

This book was written in a spirit of optimism and energy. I cannot claim that it will change your life, but perhaps it will provide some of the ammunition to help you change it for yourself. The book takes a long, hard look at what it is like to be large, weighs up the pros and cons and suggests some possible strategies to help you achieve a more positive self-image and a better quality of life.

The object is not to persuade you that you should be fat or thin, but that you should be whatever size feels natural and healthy for you. This does not, of course, mean that you should ignore the fact that being *very* overweight can have serious medical complications. Yet recent research suggests that moderate obesity, at least in women, poses no great risks to health and that it is often the stress of having a poor self-image which poses the biggest risk of all.

My book is neither for nor against diets. It is a source-book to help you make your own informed choice. Although you should always consult your general practitioner when you are planning changes in your lifestyle, you are the only person with the right to decide how you should live or how much you will weigh. And remember, dieting is hardly likely to succeed if you're only doing it to please somebody else.

The main focus of the book is on women, because they were the people who came forward to talk to me and urged me to set out their hopes, fears and experiences for others to read. Up to now, it is women who have led the 'fat liberation' movement in this country, and there has been little attempt to bring men's issues into the public domain. However, I am in no doubt whatsoever that fat men also face formidable problems in their daily life, and that is why I have included a chapter dealing specifically with them. Many of the other chapters, and especially the self-help sections, will appeal to both male and female readers.

I interviewed dozens of big women during my research, as I felt it important that this book should not contain only my own observations, but should also provide an outlet for other points of view. Wherever possible, I have illustrated my own remarks with quotes from interviewees.

You will notice that I have used the words 'fat', 'big' and 'large' more or less interchangeably. There is no sinister purpose behind this choice of vocabulary. Some people are uncomfortable with the word 'fat', while others insist on using it all the time because they say this is the only way to reclaim it from its negative connotations. Unfortunately there is no single accepted adjective. I have tried to avoid monotony, and use a range of adjectives which appeal to as many people as possible. So as not to trivialize the issues, I have avoided euphemisms like 'chubby' and 'plump'.

No matter what size or shape your body is, the chances are that you don't regard it as perfect. We in the West have become obsessive critics of our own bodies – and other people's. We allow society to set impossibly narrow standards of 'acceptability', and then spend our lives agonizing because we don't match up to them. What a strange way to behave!

Isn't it about time we stopped punishing ourselves, and tried to put body size into perspective?

1

A Small World?
Large Women Today

They say it's a small world – ask any woman over size 14. Whether she's trying to buy a glamorous outfit or going into hospital for an operation, the large woman faces constant reminders of her 'abnormal' size.

I have always thought it rather odd that the norm should be thought of as a size 10 or 12 in a society where 59 per cent of women are a size 14 or above, and around 46 per cent are a size 16 or over. As people get bigger and broader, the range of 'acceptable' sizes gets smaller and smaller – and more of us find that we don't measure up to society's impossible standards.

What is it like to be a large woman today? Why do we put up with all the pressures and the propaganda? And can we do anything to change the attitudes that shape our lives?

Slim or go naked: the tyranny of fashion

Every large woman I have spoken to cites clothes as the number one problem. This may sound rather trivial ('if that's the worst they have to worry about, things can't be that bad'), but clothes are more than just a covering to protect your body from the elements. To thin women, clothes are a vital means of self-expression. To most large women, they are a perennial nightmare. The assistant's sneering half-smile and the phrase 'nothing in your size, Madam', are engraved on millions of despairing minds.

To quote Dr Marcia Germaine Hutchinson, 'Most ready-to-wear clothing is only ready-to-wear if you are Brooke Shields. I call this the tyranny of the fitting room, a constant reminder that we don't fit. We must change our bodies to fit into clothes, or go naked' (*Transforming Body Image*, California, The Crossing Press, pp. 23–4).

The tyranny of fashion is such that those of us who don't fit this narrow stereotype feel we are faced with an ultimatum: change your body to fit the clothes or make do with a crimplene sack. Simply by refusing to produce wearable clothes at reasonable prices and in a wide range of sizes, clothing manufacturers can ensure that the diet

1

industry continues to flourish and teenagers try to starve themselves into 'normality'.

A new decade has not brought much comfort, either. Early in 1990, the papers were full of pictures of Barbie-doll lookalike Diane Brill. Ms Brill is an American model, tipped as the 'figure of the 90s', whose 40–23–40 (100–57–100 in cm!) figure was chosen by the Adel Rootstein company as the pattern for their latest High Street display mannequins.

Diane Brill certainly has a remarkable body. Her gravity-defying hourglass curves achieve what Victorian women could only manage with the aid of a whalebone corset. Yet remarkable does not necessarily mean either desirable or realistic. A figure like Ms Brill's is just as unattainable for the thin woman as it is for the fat. As one journalist remarked, you can't buy large breasts and a well-upholstered bottom over the counter.

Gabrielle is a television researcher who is expected to take great pains with her appearance. At the age of 31, she broke her back in a riding accident and – although the bones mended in time – something inexplicable and terrifying happened to her metabolism. Within a few months, her weight had doubled to 18 stone. Ten years later, and still a large woman, she has found that clothes have changed from being a joy to being a source of disappointment and feelings of failure:

> Whenever I go shopping with friends, I'm always the one who stands outside and holds the coats. I can never find anything. There are far too many manmade materials in the larger clothes, and the racks in shops like Evans are far too close together. What's more, the changing-rooms aren't pretty like they are in 'normal' clothes shops. It's like a punishment. At somewhere like Selfridge's, a simple cotton dress will cost at least £120. It used to make me cry when people said 'Have you heard? Evans have got a sale on.'

For the large woman who does not live in a big city and has a limited budget, Evans may be the only option when it comes to buying clothes. While most of the women I spoke to appreciated the improved service that Evans has offered in recent years, there was also a great deal of anger about the general unavailability of reasonably priced, fashionable clothes in large sizes and *in ordinary shops*.

Segregation of large sizes into special shops or sections is a sore point with many large women. Although some enjoy the intimacy and privacy of a specialist shop or department, most find it acutely

2

embarrassing to be seen going into an 'outsize' shop, or walking out with an Evans carrier-bag.

As Elaine – a 46-year-old farmer's wife – points out:

> In Germany, America, Canada and Australia they have much bigger clothes in the same shops as all the others. Over here, there's still a stigma about going into Evans. They should have big clothes in ordinary department stores. If someone really got onto the fashion bandwagon, and went to town with lots of fashion shows, adverts and commercials, reactions could change completely within a few months.

Although Elaine has come to terms with her size, and makes most of her own clothes, she admits that her occasional forays to the shops for 'special' outfits are rather spoiled by the taint of discrimination. She particularly dislikes the British system of 'segregating' large-sized clothes in separate shops.

So why is it that the fashion industry refuses to produce a wide range of stylish clothes in large sizes, or to treat its large customers like everyone else by including a broad size range in all 'normal' outlets? What's more, why do large women have to settle for second-best in terms of quality as well as style? Jenny – who describes herself as 'Rubens and a bit' – complains:

> I know what I'm going to find – manky viscose two-pieces. The armholes are wrong. The skirts aren't long enough. The attitude seems to be: if you're not the norm, hard luck. . . . I think designers discriminate against big women. For example, I heard Bruce Oldfield saying on *Wogan* that he doesn't want us wearing his clothes. Why not? Does he think we'd ruin them? It's terrible trying to find anything wearable at a reasonable price. You're like the child with his nose pressed up against the sweet-shop window, feeling shabby and worse about yourself each day.

Most of us – men and women – think of Marks and Spencer as a mainstay for everyday quality clothing and underwear. Yet many of the women I spoke to complained that they can never find anything over a size 18 in M&S, despite advertisements for the much-vaunted 'Plus' range (which goes up to a size 24). I contacted Marks and Spencer only to be told that the company would rather not comment as its 'policy changes frequently and might have changed again before the book comes out'. In the meantime – while M&S consider their policy – large women scour stores up and down the country for size 24 cotton knickers and buy up the entire stock wherever they find them.

When the *Clothes Show Magazine* investigated the situation ('Sizing up the problem', February/March 1990) they encountered the same attitude. Most designers refused to comment and asked not to be mentioned: obviously the issue is a real hot potato. High street retailers Miss Selfridge explained disdainfully that producing larger-sized clothes would damage their young image and 'distort the styling'.

Next recently announced with a flourish that they were about to offer 30 per cent of mail order styles and 20 per cent of clothes in shops up to a size 18. Admittedly this is quite an advance for a company which a couple of years ago insisted that it did not want a 'freak section' in its shops. But why such a small proportion of styles? Next claim that 'It is a question of offering larger sizes in the designs that can take it.' Unfortunately, this means that once again, larger-than-average women are told which styles they may wear and which ones 'will not suit them'.

There is a fundamental error in the fashion industry's assumption that size 16 is huge, massive, abnormal; and that extending a range to include size 18 is a charitable gesture in favour of shapeless social misfits who don't deserve to wear nice clothes anyway. Presumably they expect to make a big profit, or they wouldn't do it at all. Are they hoping that if they deprive large women of fashionable clothes they will eventually get the message, become thin, and conform?

But of course, size 16 is hardly large at all. During a recent TVam feature on fashions for the over-50s, the resident fashion expert commented that she had covered 'all shapes and sizes'. Her models in fact ranged from size 10 to a very compact size 14. And if the fashion industry thinks *that* is enormous, what hope for a size 26 or 30?

Totally committed to addressing the problem are Helen Teague and Rita Jarvis, otherwise known as 'Big Clothes'. Their tiny, crowded shop in North London has been trading for several years now and they have hundreds of regular customers and mail-order clients.

Helen explains the secret of their success:

> We do trendy, fashionable clothes such as leggings and big T shirts – and assuming you like our style, there are no limits on how you can dress. Our range is no brighter or more colourful than the range in any ordinary shop, but we are giving many big women their first chance to develop their own style. . . . Our customers are ordinary people, not ultra-modern – and range in age from

around 12 to 80. We offer sizes small, medium and large, starting at size 18, plus a few extra-large garments so that the really big customer will always have something. We've never had a customer we couldn't help. We find that many ladies are delighted to find that they take a 'small' or a 'medium', whereas before they have always been classed as 'outsize'.

According to Helen, having access to stylish clothes can make all the difference to a big woman's life: 'A lot of our customers change when they get access to really comfortable, fashionable clothes. They develop their own self-image. They change their jobs, chuck out their men and don't lie down and take so much any more.'

Although specialist shops like Big Clothes are beginning to appear all over the country, and some high street shops (such as Etam) are moving into wider size ranges, they still represent a tiny fraction of the service demanded by large women in Britain.

Many people have been on holiday to America and come back full of praise for the changes which are happening over there, and anger for the slow pace of change in this country. Although the situation in the United States is far from perfect, specialist magazines like *Radiance* and *Big Beautiful Woman* have brought 'queen-size' fashion into the public eye. Through their wide-ranging coverage of important issues, they have shown that large women can be fit, intelligent, beautiful *and* fashion-conscious. The fact that they also represent a huge fund of untapped spending power has not gone unnoticed by American manufacturers.

How long before shops like Big Clothes stop being the exception and start becoming the norm?

Taking up space – social life, access and public provision

Simple activities like getting onto a bus can be difficult for anyone who is larger than the 'average'. It can be a nightmare for anyone who suffers from a physical illness or disability and also happens to be large. Just going out for the evening with friends can be difficult if you are not thick-skinned, since the general public seem to think they have a right to make comments and snigger at body shape and size.

Heather Smith is a founder-member of the London Fat Women's Group, set up as a support-group for large women who are tired of apologizing for their size and who wanted to set about changing attitudes. She is fat herself, and knows how alienated other fat women can feel: 'many . . . are agoraphobic because they don't feel they deserve to exist or be seen in public spaces, and because of the extreme levels of abuse many fat women experience every time they move down a street, enter a pub, club or restaurant' (writing in the radical feminist magazine *Trouble and Strife* 16, Summer 1989).

Fellow group member Diana Pollard agrees, but feels that the problems faced by large women can be classified into two types:

> I think there is a significant difference between what society calls fat (that is, absolutely any female who has any flesh on her bones whatsoever) and my own feeling, which is '90 kg (200 lb) plus' – the women who don't go to the theatre because they simply don't fit at all. The women who don't have access to a whole range of things that other women have access to. Women who are *considered* fat do suffer – in relationships, in terms of getting 'front-of-house' jobs etc – but in terms of access they don't have the same problems.

Undoubtedly there are problems for any person – male or female – whose body cannot fit comfortably into an aeroplane toilet or a theatre seat; but is there a satisfactory solution? The London Fat Women's Group stress the need to make better provision for large people, yet others fear that this might in itself be a form of discrimination. Imagine the humiliation, they point out, of being segregated from the rest of a theatre audience in the 'fat people's seats'.

Yet something surely has to be done. McDonalds do not have to have fixed seating in their burger bars. Public toilets could be made more spacious. Seats on trains and buses could be better designed and made more comfortable for *all* passengers. As long as the world is full of these unnatural obstacles, they will stand as a silent reproach to the large man or woman who feels excluded from living a normal life. The implication will continue to be: 'You're fat so you should be ashamed of yourself. Hide yourself away and don't come out until you're thin.'

Lee works as a telephonist and is also a freelance writer, model and cartoonist. She is 42 and a size 26. Despite her many accomplishments, Lee feels excluded by the world around her: 'I have certainly been frightened by turnstiles, the new Tube barriers, and embarrassed by car and plane seat belts, and sometimes seats. I often feel sheepish about taking up more than my fair share of space. My size is a daily torment to me.'

The situation calls for a radical rethink. If we adapt public provision it must be with everyone in mind, not just fat people. We have to get away from the mythical notion of the 'normal' person, and think in terms of making amenities user-friendly for everyone – the fat, the thin, the tall, the short, the young and the old, the disabled and the ablebodied. The tall man who cannot fit into his car and the young mother who has to negotiate a double buggy around a town centre have an equal right to consideration. The question is: are *we* equal to the challenge and do we want to be?

Just desserts – fat women and food

The relationship between large women and food is a complex one. The health consequences of diets are discussed later (in Chapter 5); here we shall look at some of the disturbing social implications of food for the fat woman.

Society's assumption is that fat people are gluttons, and that this is the only reason why they are fat. So the act of eating becomes a guilty one, particularly for women – who are expected to be slender and 'in control'. Ironically, whereas society assumes that fat women love to 'pig out', to stuff themselves with food, the reality is that many large women are afraid to eat at all, especially in public. To be seen eating anything other than a lettuce leaf is to provoke the barbed comment: 'Eating again?'

According to actress Annette Badland:

When you're on a diet your whole day is geared around food. You're either feeling naughty or feeling virtuous. You get to mid-morning and you ask yourself: 'shall I eat this biscuit with my coffee? Shall I save it for later? Am I allowed to eat anything at all? Dare I be seen eating?' Food dominates your day. I remember being at a buffet once, eating no more than anyone else. Someone said 'Ooh, you'll get fat!' So I clenched my teeth and said 'Well it won't show, will it?'

It seems that fat women do not deserve to eat. The only way in which they can gain some degree of approval is to be seen to be on a permanent diet. Thin people all too often forget that individuals can have very different metabolic rates. There are women who can eat no more than a few hundred calories per day without putting on weight. Yet thin people assume that if the fat woman ate moderately, she would be as thin as they are.

Diana Pollard points out that even when it is trying to be compassionate, society does little more than patronize:

> The assumption is that every fat woman has an eating disorder, that she's a compulsive eater or eats all the wrong foods. People say 'If you ate properly, you wouldn't be fat'. Most fat people know that just isn't true, to their cost. It's quite possible to eat healthily and moderately and still be fat. And of course crash dieters – who keep their weight artificially low – are often people who eat very badly. Yet they are praised for their 'self-control'.

Of course, some fat women do suffer from eating disorders. So do a lot of thin women. The most 'successful' anorexics and bulimics are not fat. Either way, the chances are that their obsession with food has a lot to do with the pressures placed upon them by society to make them diet. Recent medical research suggests that women do not generally get eating disorders until they have discovered the pleasures and pain of dieting.

So the fat woman who is happy with the shape she is and hates lettuce has to face the glares or pitying looks of those around her as she eats or drinks – *whatever* and *whenever* she eats and drinks. Some women dread eating a packed lunch at work: 'Eating again, dear?' – the inevitable chorus of disapproval from her thin colleagues whose lives consist of endless dieting and deprivation. You just know they are thinking 'I starve myself and suffer to look like this – why the hell shouldn't you suffer too? How dare you be fat and happy? If you gorge yourself, you should take the consequences.'

But relatively few large women *do* gorge themselves. Jenny (a size 24–26) is furious at the raised eyebrows and loaded remarks:

> Those of us who are constantly fighting our bodies get no sympathy at all. If you go into a pub and treat yourself to a gin and tonic and a bag of crisps, someone will say 'Eating again?' That might be the only food you've had all day. I really don't see why we should have to apologize.

TV researcher Gabrielle agrees. Pressures from friends and colleagues to lose weight have destroyed food as an important point of social contact for her. She is reluctant to accept dinner invitations, and if forced to do so she always takes her own calorie-counted meal with her. She is terrified of accidentally eating 'more than she should'. She explains: 'I do like food, but I'm so disciplined now that I find it terribly difficult to eat anything I shouldn't. I don't even enjoy food very much any more.'

Times are changing, and large women are beginning to realize that society has been brainwashing them into feeling guilty. Food is not just a source of fuel for our bodies: it also gives us social contact and physical pleasure. It can't be natural for every mouthful to be seasoned with guilt.

Already, in America, the barriers are beginning to come down. There the National Association to Advance Fat Acceptance (NAAFA) has been working since 1969 to give fat people the right to ordinary lives and ordinary pleasures. To NAAFA, the punitive atmosphere surrounding fat people and food is simply another manifestation of 'fat oppression'.

Radiance, a successful American magazine for large women, has worked hard to banish the old taboos about fat women and food. The message put forward in the magazine's 'Voluptuous Gourmet' column is that good, wholesome food is a pleasure which all people should enjoy, *whatever* their size. A dislike or fear of food is just as unhealthy as obsessive eating.

What matters, ultimately, is that fat people should allow themselves the pleasures of cooking, eating and socializing. Refusing to give dinner-parties for your friends, simply because you are not thin, is a meaningless and self-inflicted punishment. Learning to live comfortably and naturally with food is a part of learning to live with your size. Habitually depriving yourself of all the foods you enjoy deepens a food obsession rather than cures it.

To put it another way – and borrowing a phrase from an American lapel badge – 'fat people deserve dessert'.

Thin girls don't get ill – doctors and discrimination

Physicians are . . . unsympathetic. They find fat patients distasteful. Fat people seem more difficult to examine, less likely to cooperate. Fat people are waddling reminders of the failure of medicine to come to a safe, workable program for long-term weight reduction, just as poor people and homeless people are stark reminders of the failure of the economic system. Like politicians, physicians blame the victims (Hillel Schwartz, *Never Satisfied*, reviewed in *Radiance*, Summer 1987).

Not all doctors dislike or discriminate against fat patients, but the view expressed above fits in well with the experiences of many of the women I talked to. One told me that a gynaecologist had prescribed hormones for her. 'I'd rather not,' she said. 'I've heard they have side-effects.' 'Oh, well, you might put on weight,' he replied. 'But you're fat already, aren't you?'

Jenny evokes the sense of being in jail which many fat women experience when they go into hospital: 'Straight away out comes the pink sticker: "Obesity Diet". It's taking away your ability to control what you put in your mouth. It's like being treated as a naughty child.'

Being fat is a good excuse for doctors to treat their patients badly. In many cases they have been trained to look upon obesity as a selfinflicted problem, a weakness – almost a form of suicide. They have been trained to think of fat as the inevitable harbinger of disease, without exception. Since doctors are human beings, they are also subject to the general social prejudice against big people. Many take advantage of their patients' poor self-image to make them feel even worse.

Diana Pollard recalls the case of a friend who was taken into hospital and starved under strict medical supervision. She lost no weight. The doctors accused her of cheating. They observed her even more strictly. She still lost virtually no weight. They were amazed:

> But instead of helping her to become a fit fat person, they offered her an intestinal bypass operation. It's so negative. I would like to see the medical profession accept that there is a wide range of body weights and that, regardless of your weight, it is important to exercise safely and properly for your age, weight and ability, and to eat the right things. . . . Inevitably, many women receive no medical help because they are treated so badly that they refuse it, or because they are told 'we won't take your illness seriously until you've lost weight.' I even met one 9½ stone woman whose doctor told her 'you've only got arthritis because you're so fat'.

In Chapter 5 we discuss the question of whether it is possible to be fat *and* healthy, and how to cope with a discriminating doctor.

Good girls get good jobs – large women and work

During its brief lifespan, the British magazine *Extra Special* helped many large women to take great strides forward in self-acceptance. Billed as a magazine for ladies of size 16 and above, *ES* was launched in 1987. It was immediately welcomed with open arms by millions of women desperate to read something positive about themselves and their size. Even though the magazine is long gone, many women still speak fondly of it and treasure the back issues which they have saved, read and re-read again and again.

Extra Special was always in the vanguard of the movement to bring issues out into the open and so change public opinion. In the October/November 1987 issue, editor Eleanor Graham drew readers' attention to the plight of a woman who, at 80 kg (12 stone), had been refused a job because she was 'too heavy'.

A doctor who carried out many employment medicals wrote in to the magazine and put forward an argument that seems to inspire many employers in their choice of workers:

> An employer wants to be sure that the would-be employee is not going to take more than the average amount of time off sick or develop an incapacitating illness early in life and need to draw prematurely on the pension fund. There is no arguing with the statistics which find higher rates of disease in people who are much overweight. Why should an employer hire people who are not as good a risk as those of normal weight?

The key phrase here is 'much overweight'. At 80 kg (12 stone), the candidate in question was at worst plump, and many would say healthily sturdy. There is *no* satisfactory evidence linking moderate heaviness with – say – premature death. Also, in a job involving physical strength and stamina a large, fit body is surely more useful to an employer than an artificially skinny, half-starved frame.

This may be the truth, but many employers are reluctant to admit it. It is convenient to play on the health angle, because that excuses them from admitting the real reason why they don't like employing large women: namely looks. If you don't fit into the corporate image, you're simply not going to get the top jobs.

Look at advertising. It doesn't matter how talented you may be – if you are also fat you are very unlikely to get a job, because of the client contact involved. The agency is seeking to project an image consisting of various elements: youthfulness, dynamism, efficiency . . . and slenderness. A fat creative director might evoke negative emotions in a client.

Look at any office equipment magazine. All the advertisements are peopled by willowy, glamorous females who look more like fashion accessories than efficient members of staff. Even slim secretaries get hot under the collar (and rightly so) about the media image of their profession – and it's much, much worse for the fat would-be secretary.

On 15 December 1988, the *Daily Star* carried a story headlined 'Shrink op saved me: the 24-stone hulk who became a slimline beauty.' This told the story of Shirley, a girl who resorted to dangerous intestinal surgery because of pressure from doctors and employers. She could not get a job because of her size, even though she was a fully trained secretary.

In desperation, she asked her mother to get her a job at the local cinema where she worked as an usherette, but even in the darkness her size caught up with her: 'One of the worst moments of my life was when the manager asked my mum to keep me out of sight of the customers because I looked so awful. That sort of comment can cripple a young girl.'

Cathy Smith works as an account executive in the London offices of a French bank. I asked her if she'd prefer me to quote her anonymously, but she said 'No: use my name. I'll send a copy of the book to my employers!'

A size 20–22 and 1.7 m (5′7″), Cathy has lived and worked overseas and has never encountered any prejudice . . . except in Britain. She now feels that she is being prevented from doing her job properly:

> I am now being told that I cannot visit my clients unless I get thin. Talk about discrimination. Some of my male colleagues are overweight, rarely wash – but they can visit anyone they like! It makes me so angry. I am seriously considering a change of job, but find my self-confidence has deserted me. What a cruel and ugly world.

But there is another side to the story. Not every fat woman is hampered by her size, and a positive self-image can do wonders to demolish the prejudices of employers. Others take an alternative route: self-employment.

Diana Pollard and Barbara Shores found that self-employment was the perfect solution to the problems they had encountered in the world of work. Diana explains:

> Barbara and I are entrepreneurial-type people. As fat women, we've both always thought that if you're going to do anything interesting in this world, you'll have to set it up yourself. Most people have such standard ideas of what you must look like if you're going to work for them. . . . Barbara manages a rock band, which is very unusual: everyone's anorexic in the pop world! We're both fairly dynamic. I do catering consultancy work, and a lot of

what I do is actually giving advice on nutrition. People are sometimes surprised to see a fat woman putting together balanced menus for people and getting them to introduce healthier eating into their canteens.

Self-employment has certainly worked for Barbara and Diana, and they have now embarked on a joint venture, setting up Rotunda, Britain's first fat women's press. Through this medium, they hope to get positive images of fat women out of the closet and onto British bookshelves. They are very determined women, and will probably succeed.

But we are not all cut out to work for ourselves – nor should we feel that we have to, just because we are not thin. The only permanent solution is for large women everywhere to band together and work to change employers' attitudes. Then they may finally gain access to the jobs for which they have trained and which are theirs by right.

Fat pride versus prejudice – monsters, myths and discrimination

It can be tough trying to feel good about yourself when – by society's narrow standards – your body is unacceptable. A recent survey by *What Diet and Lifestyle* (October/November 1989) produced the following depressing results:

Do you think that fat people are discriminated against?	Yes (86 per cent)
Do you think overweight women are more discriminated against than overweight men?	Yes (79 per cent)
Do you feel that potential employers are likely to favour a slim job candidate?	Yes (86 per cent)

In the survey 24 per cent believed that overweight women were treated less favourably in hotels and restaurants, 31 per cent that doctors exercised discrimination, and a massive 87 per cent complained about the treatment of large women in dress shops.

Only 38 per cent of the women said they were basically happy with their bodies, and 39 per cent hoped to have cosmetic surgery. When asked to rate their bodies on a scale of 1 to 10, three-quarters rated themselves 6 or under. To quote the magazine, 'Given one wish, the survey respondents would pick a beautiful body over a brilliant brain

– but the majority would rather have a million pounds. Perhaps to buy a better body?'

The article ends by asking: 'Isn't it time we stopped judging people by the way they look?', a fine sentiment, but a little hollow coming from a magazine whose models are always slim and attractive. At any rate, it looks as if we still have a long way to go.

Beaten by the beauty trap?

In our society, women are very much at the mercy of what Nancy C. Baker has called 'the beauty trap'. In order to gain approval, we must first achieve a particular type and level of physical appearance. If we fail to do so, we may very quickly begin to believe that we are 'not worthy' of having relationships, or that we 'don't deserve' nice clothes.

As Anna Knowles noted in *Extra Special*:

> Self-control in our society has come to mean only one thing: controlling your appetite for food. Manage that and there is no need to control the greed for possessions, status and money which is far more damaging to human relationships, civilized values – and starving people – than a big bust or plump hips.

All too often, the obsessive desire for 'perfection' leads to anorexia which (ironically) makes the sufferer far less physically attractive.

A satirist once said: 'To man, a man is but a mind. Who cares what face he carries or what clothes he wears? But a woman's body is the woman.' This may be a simplistic view – after all, in today's fitness-conscious society men face considerable pressures to change their bodies, too – but many women will recognize the truth about a woman being judged solely by her appearance. The mere sight of a large woman provokes some people into tirades of abuse, gales of laughter or humiliating sarcasm. But why such antipathy to fat women? What have we done to deserve such playground bullying?

Health education officer Liz Swinden is a size 20–22 and knows all about the prejudice affecting large women. It drives her mad:

> The trouble is the ideal woman regarded by our society is so thin that women of all sizes are pressurized into thinking they should lose weight. Fat ones are treated as an aberration, a joke – lazy, dirty, greedy, stupid and out of control. Everyone feels they have a

right to tell you what to do with yourself. Total strangers at bus-stops tell me it's a pity I'm so fat when I've got such a nice face.

It's not just a case of men cat-calling from building sites, either. Often the reaction from other women can be even more unpleasant. In fact, women are often their own worst enemies. Look at their reluctance to abandon their corsets. When it comes to body size they are just as bad. Women frequently take an 'I'm-suffering-so-why-can't-you?' attitude. According to Annette Badland: 'I think it frightens them that they could be fat too. There's some seed of fear there. They assume that we eat masses and are still jolly, and they resent it.'

Jamaican poet James Berry agrees:

My own observation is that other women detest large women. I think generally they are seen as careless and slovenly and letting down the female sex. From time to time I've heard women getting really angry with an overweight woman and saying 'Why don't you lose weight?' They talk about them behind their backs.

So why accept this ideal of artificial slenderness in the first place? According to the London Fat Women's Group, it all has a lot to do with the stereotypes put forward by the media – the Princess Diana figure, the relentless criticism of fat people by Lynda Lee-Potter and Nina Myskow, the 'Dynasty' corporate image with which television and films bombard us night after night.

Thin has become associated with young, successful and rich – values towards which we are all encouraged to aspire. The image is all-important, and can only be gained through 'control' – according to Helen Teague (of Big Clothes), the issue of control is at the heart of society's dislike of fat women: 'I think it's a fundamental issue of power, and that women are encouraged to remain small, powerless, like children. People really do seem to overreact to the idea of big women – they find it threatening to male patriarchal power.'

Indeed they do overreact. But the snag is that women are naturally fatter than men. Their bodies are intended to contain a higher proportion of fat. Hormones and the process of pregnancy tend to encourage the laying down of body fat. So for most of us, the 'corporate' body is also an unnatural one.

Suffer the little children

Even in childhood, fat carries an immense stigma. In fact, studies have shown that parents pass on their negative attitudes to their children at a very early age. Many of the women I spoke to recalled with pain the humiliation they had endured as young girls, leading on to the endless slimming treadmill and a string of failed diets:

> When I was 17 and only a size 14, a cousin said 'You're a fine stout girl, aren't you?' I was mortified. I went on a diet (Jenny).
>
> I felt like Mae West in the land of the Munchkins. . . . I ran from the burdens of womanhood and hid in the cookie jar. (Ann Harper, *The Big Beauty Book*).

The BBC television programme *QED* recently presented a documentary on Camp Shane – a summer camp for overweight children in the Catskill Mountains, USA. Parents from all over America save hard to raise over £2000 to send their children to a nine-week summer camp at which their children will be dieted and exercised – they hope – into slender conformity. ('Welcome to fat camp', 7 February 1990).

Some of the children come unwillingly ('I've been telling my mother for ten months that I didn't want to come, and she still sent me'), while others who are perfectly slim actually beg their parents to send them. Take this disturbing statement by Melissa, a cheerleader: 'I don't want to be looked at as not fat. I want to be looked at as thin. Another 6 kg (12 lbs) and I'll be perfect. I'll be so happy.' Melissa failed to lose the weight, and – a few months later – was fatter than she had been to start with.

Nevertheless, it is not difficult to see the appeal of the camp for children who are very large and who suffer from bullying and discrimination. Some of the 'guests' came along out of desperation, unable to bear the criticism any more. By no means all were girls. Josiah had already reached breaking point within himself:

> When you walk down the street there are people you don't even know. They just pass by you and look at you as though you're something from another planet. Or they call you an ape and it just hurts. . . . And after a while, after fourteen years, you can't take it any more. I really don't care whether I'm fat or skinny, just as long as I'm normal. When you're normal there's nothing wrong with you. When you're not, it's like you exist only for the normal people, just so that they have something to laugh at or something so they can say 'God, I'm sure lucky that I'm not that person'. You

16

have to stop and think. When you *are* that person, it's not that easy at all.

Josiah's decision to try to lose weight was his own. Yet others were bullied into coming by parents who were worried about their 'unacceptable' appearance but unwilling to take the time to help their children in the home environment. Do we have the right to make children suffer for their size in a world more full of junk food than love?

Fat, friends and lovers – relationships and body size

For most women, becoming fat is something dark and frightening. To sympathize with a fat woman is in some way to ally yourself with her fatness, to become associated with it – and perhaps even to risk becoming fat yourself. To be the friend or lover of a fat man or woman is a taxing experience even for the strong.

My fat friend

Many large women have excellent and enduring friendships with men and women of all sizes. But a significant minority find that their size has an unfortunate effect on the way potential friends and acquaintances see them. Lee explains:

Most men see me as asexual. Women know I am 'no threat' and tend to patronize. Friends often annoy with diet tips etc. Petite 'girlie' types sometimes attach themselves to me, although we have little in common – to 'set off' their own cuteness and appeal? I also find I get on well with gay men, whose humour I enjoy: the 'no threat' syndrome again, perhaps?

Quite a number of large women find themselves cast in the role of 'mother confessor' or sister figure. This is all very well up to a point, but there are times when the large woman also has problems and feelings that she wishes to share. It's destructive to allow other people to ignore the inner you – so practise telling them to go away sometimes.

A good rule is *never* to accept friendships that are based on the desire to humiliate or use you. I know that sounds impossible, but it isn't. If you are settling for this type of relationship it is because you undervalue yourself and others sense this. Once you begin to show that you respect yourself, others will follow suit.

17

Sadly, large women often go to great lengths not to get together. Only too often two large women at a gathering will eye each other from a distance and avoid meeting. To be seen together would be an acknowledgement that they were both fat. This makes it very difficult to achieve any sort of dialogue. Have the courage to share your feelings – good and bad – with other large women and you will all benefit from the experience.

A love that dare not speak its name?

I think a lot of men find fat fat women attractive, but they're afraid of that. Fat women need to support each other, yet women are brought up to be competitive and nasty. I think anyone who has a fat person for a lover has enormous societal pressure to try and obtain the price of that love, which is that you now become a thin person: 'I do love you – that should help you lose weight' (Diana).

Poet James Berry comes from Jamaica, where there is no discrimination against fat women – in fact they are seen as highly desirable. Nevertheless, he admits to being influenced by western standards:

I think that I have a sexual emotion for large women – for large-bosomed, bottomed and thighed women. But I must also say that there is this thing in me which wants to apply the double standard, which would want the girl that I walk out with to be nice and slim and elegant. But I do have this sexual drive for the big woman. I think many European men also find the more luscious woman sexually attractive – it's an extraordinarily instinctive thing.

The 'threat/no threat' syndrome is an interesting one. First of all, a fat woman may be a threat to a man because her body is an exaggerated representation of her sexuality. On the other hand some would say she is no threat because men are taught to regard only thin women as high-status girlfriends. Who could possibly want to go out with a fat girl? My husband's safe with her.

This view of the large woman as asexual is completely erroneous. As James Berry points out, many men are attracted specifically to large women. A dating agency – Plump Partners – has been set up to cater for those who are particularly seeking a large partner. Others are attracted to individual women, who may or may not be large – it doesn't really matter. To quote John (who is himself 'medium large' and married to a large lady):

> Far better a fat intelligent pleasant woman than a thin moron! I've no real hang-up about big women, and I'm sceptical about mother-figure theories. Who cares? It's what's between the ears that counts, not the weight. After all, in Saudi Arabia, I'd be a pin-up!

Anthony is 40 and works as a journalist. Nowadays, he makes no secret of his appreciation of large women; but his attitude wasn't always so relaxed, as he explains:

> I think it's a great shame – this tyranny of fashion. I've always been a great admirer of larger ladies, though I think it's something that's got more pronounced with age.
>
> When I was in my teens and early twenties, I was much more aware of peer-group pressure. I think most young men are heavily influenced by what their friends think about them – and this doesn't just relate to music or clothes but to the type of women they go out with.
>
> Mind you, in those days (the late 1960s) although the 'Twiggy' look was supposed to be in, I don't recall any of my friends actually having a stated preference for stick-like women. We were so full of adolescent anxieties that the only thing we really worried about was whether or not we would get a girlfriend at all!
>
> I think fashion and life became infinitely more conformist in the 1980s than at any other time I can recall. We're all obsessed with our lifestyles. I personally never noticed any specific prejudice against fat until the 1980s. It's so bad now that even I am advised to slim by well-meaning colleagues (I'm 1.8 m (5'8″) and weight around 80 kg (13 stone).

Anthony believes that in some ways women are their own worst enemies:

> Women usually impose diets on themselves. It doesn't come primarily from men at all. The worst, or the most insistent, criticism of women's bodies is to be found in the pages of women's magazines. In the race to compete with men, there is an implication that perfection is a slender, masculine physique. I think that what many women perceive to be faults – say a large bottom or large thighs – men frequently find attractive.

19

As I've got older, my tastes have matured and I've become less reluctant to express my preferences. I am a lot less critical of a woman's physique. I don't expect a woman to look like Kylie Minogue. Mind you, I don't look much like Jason Donovan either! But I suppose there will always be some older men who remain Peter Pans, hankering after their lost youth.

In an article in *Radiance* (Summer/Fall 1986: 'Fat Admirers: problem or solution?') Dan Davis – a self-proclaimed 'fat admirer' examines men's attitudes towards large women, and large women's reactions to the men who are attracted to them. According to Mr Davis 'fat admirers . . . make up about 5 per cent of the male population, and we have two characteristics in common: we love fat women, and we're all but invisible to the media.'

Dan Davis, like John, dismisses 'mother figure' theories: 'most of us simply feel the same sensual attraction to the curves and softness of fat women that other men feel for the lean lines of beauty contestants'. He goes on to point out that not all men who are attracted to large women take the same uninhibited attitude towards their attraction:

> There are many more hiding in the closet. . . . Fat admirers who deny their preferences to themselves can be very unpleasant. Unable to accept their attraction to women their buddies might not approve of, they are also unable to suppress their fascination, which in turn emerges as hostility. Many of the louts who insult large women in public fall into this category. Some even marry fat women and then make their wives miserable by hounding them about their weight. Some . . . love to spend time at home with fat women but go to great lengths to avoid taking them out in public. . . .

The major problem, according to Dan Davis, is women's own insecurities. They are so sure that their admirers are only 'settling for second best' that they withdraw and become extremely difficult to approach. They think 'Why me? Men don't fancy fat women.' So the man who does set his heart on a large lady sets himself a hard task.

The main thing, in all relationships, is to value yourself. Whatever your lifestyle, there's one person you have to live peacefully with: yourself.

Big, fat and worthless? – culpability and self-image

When we look at all the problems and prejudice which large people – and women in particular – have to face, it is hardly surprising that many see themselves as guilty and worthless.

Monica's feelings are typical of many large women: 'I feel I have gone downhill quite a lot, let myself down. I suppose I'm living with guilt. I'm ashamed because I'm undisciplined. I know my husband would like me to look better.'

Some of us fall into the trap of thinking that we are only fat temporarily. We're working on it. Soon we'll be thin again and then everything will be all right. But until then we've put our lives on hold. This is a terrible punishment to inflict on yourself. You have done nothing to be ashamed of, so why should you reduce the scope and quality of your life just to satisfy other people who think you ought to feel guilty? In the words of Ruthanne Olds: 'When I was fat, I always felt it was a waste to invest in nice things. . . . We think we're just fat temporarily' (*Big and Beautiful*).

Yet this attitude is a dangerous one. While we may not all want to share the American 'fat is fantastic' philosophy, most of us are capable of feeling good about ourselves, of knowing that what we are is not just a collection of fat cells but a person with a right to feelings, thoughts and needs.

Judged, but not guilty?

I talked to many women in the course of my researches. Body size is an emotive subject, particularly for women, and news travelled fast. Some told their friends and relatives, who rang or wrote to me to ask how they could contribute their feelings and opinions to the project. The following account is taken from a letter I received. I think Mary's story describes very vividly the problems, pain and prejudice which so many large women have to face:

> I have been large ever since I can remember, on and off diets of all kinds since about age twelve. I even tried the notorious Cambridge Diet, but after eating nothing at all for four days and feeling like a social leper, I canned the diet, chucked £25 away – and promptly put back the 5 kg (10 lbs) I'd lost. Nowadays I'd love to be a size 10 or 12 (my ideal would be to be 1.5 m (5'2") tall, 34–24–34) but I daren't diet, as I'm convinced the reason I put on 30 kg (5 stone) in the last ten years is because I've mucked about with my metabolism by keeping on dieting then not dieting. I sometimes wish I lived in Tonga, where fat is beautiful!

Do you remember during the 1970s there seemed to be a spate of songs with 'fat' in them? I have a particularly cringe-making memory of being in the car with my Uncle Simon and cousin Geoff (whom I fancied something rotten then) – and that blasted song 'Hey fatty boom boom' came on the radio. Uncle Simon sang along to it, while I went redder and redder in the back seat, and when he got to the bit 'It's not because you're so big and fat; I don't believe I'm afraid of that', I thought I would die of embarrassment. I'll never, ever forget it.

I remember going to a harvest supper with my (then) new husband, as his father was the vicar there, and lining up at the cold table with our plates – something I've always hated, as you get used to people watching you like hawks to see how much you put on your plate. Anyway, the local butcher was serving the meat, and when it came to my turn he looked me up and down, winked at the other people in the queue and said 'a growing girl like you needs feeding up' – and gave me an extra slice. I was mortified. To this day, I wish I'd had the guts to ask him if he was that rude to everyone or was I a special case?

When I had bronchitis, the only way I could get to the doctor's was on the back of my husband's motor bike. I was wearing an old camouflage jacket of his, as I couldn't find proper biking gear in my size. By the time I got there, after being blasted with icy air, I was really gasping for breath. The doctor was not sympathetic. Personally I think he should have been, as we'd asked him to come out to us and he'd refused. Instead, he said the only reason I had bronchitis was because I was overweight, and if he was me, he'd want to camouflage his body, too. I think he should have been struck off for making remarks like that, but at twenty I was too meek even to retaliate verbally. Ironically, at that time I was only a size 20 and weighed 13 stone, which now seems wonderful to me! I wish I was that 'small' now.

I do *know* the philosophy I should be striving for, which is that I'm me, whatever my size, and being fat shouldn't stop me from having fun and doing whatever I want to – but it DOES. I am 'unable' to go swimming or horseriding, for instance – things I used to get a lot of pleasure from when I was a child, and both given up when I became the butt of everyone's jokes. I long to wear a bikini, but of course that's out.

Last year I flew for the first time, which I really loved, but I shan't fly again, as I suffered the humiliation of having a bum bigger than the gap between the armrests. I wonder if it was a smaller-than-normal seat, as it *was* a cheap flight, on one of those air buses, but after suffering similarly in my local cinema, now I'm not so sure. I LOVE the theatre, but now each time I visit a new one, I panic beforehand in case the seats are too small and I'm humiliated in front of my friends.

When I stayed with my sister in Paris this year, I couldn't believe how everyone stared at me, like I was a freak or something. I took to keeping my coat on in the end, although it was far too hot and sticky. I'm now planning another trip with my mum, this time by train and ferry. My mum is another large lady, and the first thing she said was 'Well, I suppose I'd better lose 25 kg (4 stone) quickly then – they're all so chic over there'. She won't of course (she's a failed dieter like me) but it's interesting that out of everything she could be looking forward to on her first trip to Paris, it's other people's rudeness.

I know I should lose weight, as I'm getting varicose veins plus I have osteochondritis in one knee and if I was half my weight, it would be half the stress on my joints. I know all this, but I do nothing. Incidentally, the only thing that's ever come close to making me feel better about myself was that wonderful magazine *Extra Special*. Unfortunately, I'd only discovered it for four issues when it ceased to be. I felt like crying.

Although I feel persecuted by society in general, I don't think it's necessarily prejudice against fat people, more prejudice against ugly people. Fat is considered ugly, hence the expression 'lose 10 lbs of ugly fat' which you see in diet ads. Those people who snigger and point the finger at me would probably do the same if I had really bad acne, or thick glasses, or facial hair, or any other little 'imperfections' from what they're told is beautiful.

I tell you, being fat in our society sucks, and people without the 'problem' have absolutely no idea of how we feel, or our needs. I hope your book pierces some consciences.

Changing things for the better

Mary's letter shows how difficult it is for a sensitive woman to lead a normal, happy life when everything seems to be conspiring to make life unpleasant for her. Practical problems like clothes and cinema seats are bad enough, but these are really only a symptom of the real problem: people's bad attitudes.

If society did not view fat as morally culpable – especially for women – then most of the practical problems would soon disappear. Instead of admitting that their failure to cater for large women is a subtle way of condemning and punishing 'excessive' body size, the powers-that-be make plausible-sounding excuses.

Dress designers say there is 'no demand' for large-size, high-fashion clothes. Doctors explain their harsh treatment of fat patients as being 'for their own good'. Employers justify their rejection of plump applicants in terms of 'risk' – yet there really is no hard evidence that a 12 stone woman will be any less healthy or efficient than one of 8 stone, and indeed she will probably be less of a 'risk' than an anorexic 6 stone girl with no strength or stamina and an unhealthy obsession with food.

Assuming we accept that these attitudes are unjustified, harsh and unfair, how do we go about changing them – without falling into the trap of implying that 'fat is good and thin is bad'?

'Fat liberation' and 'fat oppression' are well-known concepts in America, where the National Association to Advance Fat Acceptance (NAAFA) (see below) has been working to improve the quality of life for large men and women since 1969. They have less currency here in Britain, where they are more likely to raise a snigger than a nod of acknowledgement. Nevertheless, although to date little has been done over here to help fat men, a movement is afoot to help large women achieve a fuller, guilt-free life.

The struggle to be normal

There is always a danger, with any movement or pressure group, that its actions will focus public opinion on its members as 'abnormal' or 'weird'. A well-known agony aunt told me that she was opposed to the idea of this book on the grounds that 'It would be pointless to try and define people on so insignificant a detail. . . . A book such as you suggest would reinforce the idea that big people are "different". They aren't different – just big!'

There is a grain of truth in this view. Big people *aren't* different. It would be nice to think that body size really was irrelevant, that no-one ever judged us on the tautness of our bottoms or the flatness of our stomachs. Maybe one day life will be like that, but – in my opinion at least – it will take effort and many changes of heart.

NAAFA and the American dream

In America, the 'fat liberation' movement is far better established than it is here in Britain. There, fat men and women have their own national organization working for them. NAAFA (originally the National Association to Aid Fat Americans, now the National Association to Advance Fat Acceptance) was founded in 1969 by

William J. Fabrey (an electrical engineering consultant). Although specifically a North American organization, NAAFA describes its role as a 'quest for dignity, equality and happiness for large-size people throughout the world' – which has to be good news for large people in Britain, too.

It takes a multifaceted approach to the problems of being large, and offers:

- a support group for large people and their 'admirers'
- an educational function, with newsletter and other mailings
- a human rights group working for size acceptance
- computer dating and penpals
- 23 'chapters' (regional groups) in the United States and Canada
- a book service

The fact that NAAFA has grown in stature and is now in its third decade is an indication of the greater level of 'fat awareness' in America. There are many companies now offering products to make life easier for large people. It's not just a question of clothes (though these are increasingly well provided for). Amplestuff of Charlottes-ville, Virginia, for example, offer everything from large-size sculp-tures and toys to books, health products and household and car accessories. They also publish a newsletter – *Ample Shopper*. Not every large person wants to buy from specialist companies, but at least the option is there and some useful and 'fun' products are getting onto the market.

Britain catches up

Here in Britain, matters are getting off the ground at last – but slowly. At the forefront of the movement is the London Fat Women's Group, which on 18 March 1989 organized the first-ever National Fat Women's Conference at the London Women's Centre.

One of the women involved in the Conference told me why she felt it had been both important and successful (although 170 women attended, 400 other applications had to be turned away owing to lack of space and the organizers received over a thousand letters of support):

I thought it would be nice to be in a situation where I was actually surrounded by fat women – to see what it felt like. Fat women avoid each other in social situations, because it's almost like admitting they're fat. If you're fat – however long you've been fat –

it's supposed to be something you're working to get out of. So all you could talk about in that atmosphere would be dieting.

This situation is deeply problematic. To begin with, fat women cannot hope to exert much social or political influence if they avoid contact with each other. In the words of the old adage, 'United we stand, divided we fall' – and this is one of the main reasons for the creation of the London Fat Women's Group and the subsequent National Fat Women's Conference. But, quite apart from this, there is the question of isolation and psychological well-being.

Nobody is suggesting that fat women should spend all their time in the company of other fat women. Two people are not necessarily destined to become soulmates just because they share the same dress size. But by avoiding other women who have gone through similar experiences, fat women are cutting themselves off from an important source of support and encouragement. Perhaps most important of all, the fat woman who refuses to recognize her size is denying herself the chance to come to terms with it, and so release herself from some of the lifelong tensions induced by a thin-is-beautiful society.

The Conference was organized as a forum for large women to get together and talk about their problems, their hopes and fears, and to exchange opinions. It was also hoped to increase the general public's awareness of the problems and discrimination that fat women face in British society.

Needless to say, much of the media interest in the event was prurient rather than innocent. Although journalists were not allowed to take part, several tried to 'infiltrate' the conference and had to be asked to leave. There was also some trouble with press photographers who tried to take photographs of the dance workshop through the windows, and reporters who hassled women as they arrived.

Nevertheless, awareness was certainly raised. Appearances by members of the group on programmes ranging from *Wogan* to *Open Space* provoked a surge of public interest. Some jeered; many others expressed a positive interest in a subject which they had perhaps never considered before. It is easy to discount fat people if they make no noise and do not draw attention to their problems. Gabrielle, who used to be thin, admits: 'Before, I never used to think about what it must be like to be fat. I really don't know if I was prejudiced or not.'

The main issues which the Group wished to address through the Conference were health, employment, fashion and sexuality, and by the end of the day an action plan had been drawn up:

Health: a health group was set up, to lobby the NHS to provide unbiased medical research, an end to harassment and more holistic medicine; also a withdrawal of dangerous surgical procedures such as bypass surgery.

Employment: an employment group is to seek union recognition of discrimination against fat people in recruitment and of size-related harassment at work and unfair dismissal.

Fashion: a fashion group will lobby the fashion industry to improve its provision to fat women, and will challenge designers to produce clothes designed to complement a fat body. To quote Heather Smith, one of the conference organizers: 'We want to have a choice of images at prices all women can afford and we don't want to have to travel miles to buy underwear or a pair of tights.'

Other groups were also set up to address such issues as sexuality, ethnic background and the production of positive writing about fat women. It was also hoped to exert pressure on the relevant authorities to improve public provision and access. Women who attended from areas outside London were encouraged to go back to their towns and villages and set up their own support groups. Slowly but surely a network is spreading across the country.

One of the workshops produced a statement, based on an American model, which challenges many of the established assumptions about fat women. Here is an extract from it:

- Don't assume . . . I don't like my body
- Don't assume . . . I think your body is better
- Don't assume . . . You're doing me a favour by having a
  relationship with me
- Don't assume . . . I'm always happy/jolly
- Don't assume . . . I'm not sexual
- Don't assume . . . I'm single
- Don't assume . . . I'm unfit/unhealthy
- Don't assume . . . I eat more than you do
- Don't assume . . . I don't want to dance
- Don't assume . . . you look better than I do because you're thinner
- Don't assume . . . your body won't change
- Don't assume . . . I want to wear Crimplene
- Don't assume . . . I want a diet Coke
- Don't assume . . . that where you go will be accessible to me
- Don't assume . . . that my fat has psychological roots

● Don't assume . . .
   (abridged and quoted from *Fat Women's News*, Spring 1989)

Producing the statement helped members to externalize some of the pain and anger which they felt at people's assumptions about their size. The statement is also useful on a broader canvas because it presents a stark challenge to society to examine the ways in which it views fat women. Many assumptions are unspoken and inherent, rather than overt. Questions of size and sexuality, for example, are scarcely ever touched upon in polite conversation and it must come as a shock to many thin readers to recognize that they have always assumed – perhaps unconsciously – that their fat friends were not sexual beings.

This statement contains the personal feelings and observations of one group of fat women. It is not all-inclusive, and there is no reason why you should not get together with friends to produce your own version of it. Most important of all, it should be brought to the attention of the thin people you know: it could come as quite a revelation to them!

Is fat a feminist issue?

Obviously the Fat Women's Conference was organized specifically to help women – though men may benefit indirectly from some of the Group's work (for example, the battle for the abolition of the new Tube barriers, or for a more understanding attitude to fat people in general). Yet a question remains: why no London Fat *Men's* Group? In Chapter 4, we discuss society's attitudes to fat men and the problems they face.

What's it to do with me?

If you found that any of the statements above matched your own experiences of being large, you are probably wondering how we are ever going to change a collection of attitudes that have been with us for many years. More than that, you may be wondering what it all has to do with you. After all, how can one individual change the minds of millions?

Perhaps one individual can't. But hundreds or thousands of individuals, working together, can gradually chip away at the mountain until it disintegrates by, for example:

● joining (or forming) a support group, and collecting information for a local resource directory: this could contain the names of useful shops, theatres with generously proportioned seats, sympathetic doctors etc.

- getting involved in social activities or local issues (anything which enables you to show that big people are active and interesting)
- writing, phoning or turning up in person to complain – for example, to dress shops and manufacturers about the level of quality and service, the range available etc.: if you complain on your own it may not have much effect, but if you get all your friends to complain as well, you could make a real difference – use your economic power
- making the local and national press aware of the issues
- being determined to challenge hurtful or ignorant remarks and reacting with a reasoned argument to ill-informed criticism: some people even collect witty ripostes and turn the best ones into lapel badges
- telling yourself that you refuse to accept second best – ever!

Useful addresses

Big Clothes
81a Boundary Road
London NW8 0RG
Tel: 071 625 6124

London Fat Women's Group
c/o London Women's Centre
Wesley House
4 Wild Court
Holborn
London WC2

Radiance Magazine
PO Box 31703
Oakland
California 94604
USA
Tel: 415 482 0680

Big, Beautiful Woman Magazine
9171 Wilshire Boulevard
Suite 300
Beverley Hills
California 90210
USA
Tel: 213 858 0323

Rotunda Press (UK distributors of *Shadow on a Tightrope*)
PO Box 17
Glasgow
G4 9AA
Scotland

Plump Partners (introduction agency)
15 Bryn y Foel
Rhosemor
Nr Mold
Clwyd
N. Wales CH7 9PW
Tel: 0352 78091

NAAFA (National Association for Advancing Fat Acceptance)
Box 43
Bellerose
New York
NY 11426
USA
Tel: 516 352 3120

Amplestuff Ltd
1150 East Market Street
Charlottesville
VA 22901
USA

Further reading

The Beauty Trap, Nancy C. Baker (London: Piatkus, 1984)
Never Satisfied, Hillel Schwartz (New York: Free Press, 1986)
Transforming Body Image, Marcia Germaine Hutchinson (Freedom, California: Crossing Press, 1985)

A SMALL WORLD?

The Big Beauty Book, Ann Harper and Glenn Lewis (New York: Holt, Rinehart and Winston, 1982)
Big and Beautiful, Ruthanne Olds (Washington, DC: Acropolis Books, 1984)

2

Worlds of Difference:
Historical and Cultural Perspectives

How do you feel about the way you look? If you're dissatisfied, does that dissatisfaction come from within you? Is it a balanced, reasonable judgement? Or is it based on the things other people say, the articles you read and the 'perfect' people you see on TV? For most of us, body image is conditioned by a whole host of external factors, however independent we may think we are.

When we feel bad about ourselves, many of us like to daydream. We drift off in our minds to some imagined age when 'Rubens' women' were the standard for beauty and the Venus de Milo scorned corsets. Or perhaps you prefer to imagine yourself on a South Sea Island, surrounded by people who worry in case you get too thin? It's tempting to think that the best of all possible worlds is always somewhere else.

In order to put our own attitudes and feelings into perspective, it can be helpful to look at other cultures and other periods of history. From them, we can learn not only about the roots of our own body obsessions, but about other, more positive ways of looking at our bodies.

Matriarchs, patriarchs and goddesses:
body size and power

If you were to take a tape measure to the Venus de Milo, you would discover that her vital statistics are: 38–32–42 (95–80–105 cm). Even allowing for her height (1.7 m; 5'7") she is far from slender by modern standards. She could never hope to appear on the cover of *Vogue* and would have trouble finding clothes to fit her in a fashionable boutique. Exercise gurus would advise her to trim her waist and pummel the cellulite from her ample thighs. Yet she has been acknowledged for centuries as an enduring standard of beauty – the goddess of love.

Tastes change. But the tradition of the fat goddess endures. Fat gods (like Bacchus) tend to be associated with good living and prosperity. Big goddesses are symbols of feminine power and survival, of a woman's unique ability to bring forth life.

If you look at a picture of the Willendorf Venus, or look at fertility statuettes in the British Museum, you will see that they are not only pregnant: they are also very much on the plump side. These figurines

32

Chap 1 – Ideas vary

ot only have rounded bellies but
generous thighs. Every female
:gerated. Scholars have estimated
il women, the women would weigh
00 lbs; 14 to 21 stone).
that the power expressed in the
:ep-seated fears in men. When
:ss it poses a threat to patriarchal
adays want their women to be thin.
According to this theory, n are only allowed to gain power and
influence in modern society by becoming like men, by dieting until
their female characteristics are suppressed and they begin to look like
boys – hence 'power dressing'.

Interestingly, the very fat man may be seen to be emasculated by his
size. In a moderately large man, size can mean strength – but if he has
'feminine' characteristics – breasts, fat thighs, swollen belly – he may
be seen as less than a man. Extreme obesity can diminish potency in
men, and eunuchs are known to accumulate fat deposits along
feminine lines. So the very large man may appear to pose a sexual
threat to nobody.

If you find these ideas far-fetched, remember that many ethnic
groups still acknowledge the big woman as a source of strength, life
and hope for the future. For example, until recent times only a very
large woman was considered powerful enough to reign as queen in
Hawaii.

The idea makes sense when you realize that it has been strongest in
those areas of the world and periods of history where famine has been
a fact of life. To quote Paul Ernsberger, PhD, a well-known
biomedical researcher in the United States, and author of *Rethinking
Obesity* (a book which aims to change the attitudes of doctors, nurses
and other health professionals), writing in the American magazine
Radiance:

> Female obesity dates from the dawn of the Cro-Magnons, and may
> have been highly valued through much of early history. A woman
> who carried reserve food supplies on her body increased the
> chances that she and her offspring could survive on reduced rations
> for the duration of pregnancy or breast feeding under the harsh
> conditions of the Ice Age (Winter 1988, p. 34).

With such power to survive, it is little wonder that admiration often
turned to worship. These days, we may not want to be goddesses – but

we can try to regain that special sense of pride in the ample female form.

Can big be desirable?

Stop press! Perhaps you didn't realize it, but big is world news. Did you know that around 81 per cent of the world's cultures still believe that overall plumpness or moderate fatness is desirable in women? What's more, 90 per cent of cultures consider fat hips and thighs attractive. Try telling that to a model agency or the sponsors of Miss World!

Old preferences die hard, and despite vigorous efforts by public health officials in many countries, big retains its highly positive image. Take this example, quoted by Dr Ernsberger in *Radiance* magazine:

> One African poster showed a fat woman and an overloaded truck with a flat tyre; the caption read 'Both carry too much weight'. The advertisement backfired, though, because people assumed that the woman was not only wonderfully fat, but was also rich, since she had a truck weighed down with her possessions (p. 42).

Many large Westerners have wonderful tales to tell of their trips to countries where big is beautiful – not only for women but often for men too. Jane, a dress designer, tells of her trip to India:

> There were several large people in our party, and they were mobbed by the locals. The two big girls were followed around by men who wanted to marry them, and the stout, bald-headed men were very much in demand with the local girls. Why? Because big means rich! In such a poor country, only the wealthy can afford to be fat.

In countries where hunger is, or has often been, the norm, largeness is highly prized, and girls have sometimes been fattened up to make them 'fit for marriage'. In his 1923 book, *Girth Control*, Henry T. Finck adopts a suitably shocked tone of voice as he describes such customs:

> In Polynesia, the Rev W. W. Gill tells us, girls were regularly fattened and imprisoned till nightfall, when a little gentle exercise was permitted. If refractory, the guardian would whip the culprit for not eating more. To please the men, African women eat

enormous quantities of bananas and drink milk by the gallon. . . .
Mungo Park wrote that with the Moors 'corpulence and beauty are
terms nearly synonymous. A woman of even moderate pretension
must be one who cannot walk without a slave under each arm to
support her; and a perfect beauty is a load for a camel.'

Most of us today would share Mr Finck's horror at the idea of
forcefeeding girls like geese for the slaughter. But it is interesting to
see that beauty can come in many shapes and sizes, and that big is far
from ugly in many – *indeed the majority* – of cultures.

Dr G. Sobhy, an Egyptian physician writing in the late 1920s, told
of his losing battle to persuade his patients to lose weight. Nobody in
Egypt seemed to see his point of view. He pointed out that the ancient
Egyptians had made fun of fat people, but it just didn't work. As far as
his patients were concerned, big was beautiful and opulent and thin
meant hungry and poor. Dr Sobhy was particularly concerned about a
disturbing new trend that we find both peculiar and dangerous today:
'Nothing has taken in the practice of medicine in Egypt like
subcutaneous injections of arsenical compounds for fattening people.
I have often been asked by extraordinarily fat women to give them
injections of Neosal Varsan in order to make them fatter still'
(*Obesity in Egypt*).

At the other end of the scale, the poet Terence tells us that Roman
mothers were in the habit of starving their daughters to make them
reed-thin – and therefore marriageable. And an ancient book, the
Pinguis Minerva, tells us that 'If the Goddess of Wisdom were to grow
fat, even she would become stupid.' On the other hand, Greeks from
the 'decadent' period wore corsets – not to slim their waists, but to
make their hips look bigger. All in all, a confusion of attitudes that
makes our own narrow standards look equally silly.

One woman I spoke to who has learned from these widely differing
attitudes is Venus, 26 and black, born in England. At one point she
starved herself into hospital in an attempt to reduce her size 22 body
to a more 'acceptable' size 14. It wasn't until she went on a trip to
Jamaica that she realized she could be beautiful the way she was:

Over here, people will glare at a fat woman in the street. Over
there, it's no big deal. She's a big woman – so what? You see big
women in tight leggings, and tight T shirts with belts. Men will
stand and wolf whistle. I took off my T shirt and walked up and
down the beach in my swimming costume like a woman out of an
advertisement. I felt that I could achieve anything.

Jacqueline agrees with her. She spent three-and-a-half years in Sierra Leone, West Africa, as a VSO and describes them as

the happiest I've ever spent. It was all down to leaving a country where the big woman is either ridiculed or seen as 'mother earth' and living in a country where big is seen as sexy, healthy, attractive and most desirable by young and old, men and women. With tailors on every corner, I developed fashion design talents and was able to get truly stunning clothes instead of wallowing around in outsize or men's clothes. . . . Ironically, in a country where big is best where people are concerned, I lost quite a lot of weight – understandable when you consider the dire economic situation. When I returned from a holiday in Britain, everyone commented on how much stouter I was – and this was a real compliment. It makes me wonder why I bothered coming back to Britain. . . .

Does big have to be bad news?

As westernization hits developing countries and television brings images of *Dallas*-style skinnies, perceptions are slowly changing. But should they? Some scientific investigations have suggested that large people from many ethnic backgrounds may be perfectly well until they adopt a western lifestyle – and only *then* do they develop 'fat' problems like high blood pressure and heart disease.

One study was carried out in the Italian community of Roseto in Pennsylvania. Fatness was accepted in this community and plumpness was considered ideal. When the study began in the 1950s, the rate of heart attacks was less than half that in nearby towns, possibly because the residents still followed a traditional Italian diet rich in starch and low in cholesterol. During the 1960s, the traditional way of life was gradually abandoned. Diet changed . . . and along came Weight Watchers to knock them all into shape. By the mid-1970s, the heart attack rate was the same as that in the rest of Pennsylvania (see *The Roseto Story* by J. G. Bruhn and S. Wolf).

Margaret Mackenzie, a medical anthropologist, undertook a cultural study into obesity in Western Samoa. The average height of the women she studied was 1.6 m (5'4") and the average weight 90 kg (200 lbs) – very obese by western standards. Yet not one of the 101 women studied had high blood pressure, heart disease or arthritis (though a few did suffer from diabetes). Studies have since shown that when Western Samoans move to the West they become even bigger, and their children do develop dangerously high blood pressure.

Perhaps the most interesting fact in Dr Mackenzie's study is the women's own attitude to their size. They could hardly believe that anyone should want to study such a trivial issue. One woman actually confronted her:

> If I didn't want to get fat, she said, then I shouldn't get married. Because if I married, then I would get pregnant. Once I was pregnant, I would gain weight. . . . By the time I had the average six or seven children, I would be fat. That was the beginning and the end of it. And why could I not study something that was a true problem, instead of wasting so much money and effort on something so clearcut and so irrelevant? ('A cultural study . . .' *Radiance*, Summer/Fall 1986, pp. 23–25).

Fat in Western Samoa is natural, normal and unremarkable. It is something that keeps you warm and gives you energy – not a measure of moral worth, of success or of failure. That's a lesson we could all learn from.

Fat, class and culture

As we have seen, fat is far more acceptable in many other cultures than it is in the West today. Historically, it has been a mechanism for racial survival – particularly in the female, who gives birth to and nurtures the next generation and so guarantees the continuation of the family group.

If fat is such a valuable commodity, why has it ceased to be a status symbol in the West? The Tongans have long been renowned for their Royal Family – why not the British? Why are princesses expected to be willowy creatures, and not big, strong and expansive as an indication of their wealth and prestige? King Edward VII enjoyed ample proportions, so why not Prince Charles?

Recent evidence suggests that body size is closely linked with ethnic background and class. It was the Duchess of Windsor who said 'A woman can never be too rich or too thin', and indeed successful, upwardly mobile people are expected to be both.

One theory is that, as nutrition has improved in the West over the last 200 years or so, people have become generally healthier, stronger . . . and bigger. Girls begin to menstruate and develop sexual characteristics earlier, and taking the contraceptive pill increases the tendency to put on body weight.

For quite a long time now, remaining thin has been an exercise in self-torture for many people – an artificial process which is really no different from starvation. In countries where food is readily available and no-one needs to starve, going hungry has become a means of gaining kudos. In turn, it has become associated with high social standing. As early as 1923, Dr Cecil Webb-Johnson was making the point:

> Women of the British upper class are known to practise the sternest self-control in order to retain their admired slim figures. . . . Middle-aged women of the lower middle-class, whose means allows them to indulge in practically unlimited eating and drinking, often tend to become enormously stout.

His condemnation of 'undisciplined' men was no less virulent. In short, the lower down the social scale you were, the less self-discipline you possessed – which was probably why you belonged to the lower orders in the first place!

Back in 1973, research psychiatrist Maurice Yaffé came up with some interesting socioeconomic observations about obesity. He noted that, among American women, obesity was twice as prevalent in lower socioeconomic groups than in higher ones (and six times as prevalent in New York City). The trend was similar, but less pronounced, among men.

Curiously, Yaffé also reported that people tended to lose weight as they moved up the social ladder, especially if they were female. Most women will recognize that the reason for this loss of weight is almost certainly social pressure, since thinness and high social standing have become inextricably linked over the years. If you want to be really successful, it seems, you have to be rich *and* thin.

Heredity is an important causal factor in obesity. It is now agreed that, even with only one obese parent, a child stands a 40–50 per cent chance of growing up to be large. The likelihood may reach 80 per cent if both parents are big. Add to this the fact that many ethnic groups have a high tendency to put on weight, and the race to become that 'ideal', slender western shape becomes an even more ludicrous proposition.

Theories linking fat and heredity have received a recent boost from Canadian researchers led by Dr Angelo Tremblay. Twelve pairs of identical male twins, aged between 19 and 27, were confined to Laval University for 100 days. None had a history of being over-weight. During the test, each person received a daily diet containing an extra 1000 calories and was forbidden to exercise.

The results were remarkable. Pairs of twins tended to gain similar amounts of weight, but there was a marked difference between pairs. While one man gained only 4 kg (9.5 lbs), for example, another gained almost 13 kg (30 lbs). Yet all the volunteers had eaten exactly the same amount of food. Heredity was also shown to influence the way in which weight was put on, with identical twins tending to gain weight in exactly the same places.

Essentially, of course, the whole idea is ludicrous. If Lillian Russell, Lillie Langtry and Henry VIII could move in the best society, why should large people (of whatever race) be punished today for simply being what nature intended them to be?

All shapes and sizes: reshaping the body

For all their trials and tribulations, large men don't have quite the same problems with clothes as do large women. Fashions for men have changed relatively little in recent years, and are designed principally for comfort. Unfortunately that hasn't usually been the case with women's fashions.

Vagaries of fashion reflect the image of women that society wishes to convey at a given time. For example, the wasp-waist corsets of the late nineteenth century (capable of creating a perfect hourglass figure from even the most shapeless torso) and the bustles which *fin-de-siècle* ladies used to produce the fashionable 'S'-shaped outline. Crinolines, Catherine de Medici's iron corset (designed to reduce the waist to 32 cm, 13"!), the modern brassière – all of these and many more were devised to satisfy a fundamentally male desire for a certain type of woman to which so few matched up naturally – a desire which was soon perpetuated by the women themselves.

Until the 1960s, women hardly ever complained about the discomforts and inconveniences of fashionable dress. What did it matter if one's farthingale was too wide to get through the door? What if it was impossible to eat, sit down or go to the lavatory? What mattered was being considered perfect.

In the face of the nineteenth-century Healthful Dress Movement and endless medical tracts on 'corset liver', women persisted in tightlacing themselves into 'beauty' – and fainting as a result. In the case of the corset, they swallowed the moral argument hook, line and sinker. Mothers assured their daughters in the strongest terms that no respectable young lady would even sleep without a corset, let alone go out into the streets without its guarantee of physical and moral rectitude.

This type of physical reshaping is not just a feature of western society. If we look at other cultures we soon see that foot-binding, neck rings, tattooing, nose-piercing and so on are all extreme versions of the same idea. At least those traditions remained fairly constant from one generation to the next. In our society, we face continually shifting demands with which it is impossible to keep up.

We may think that bra-burning signalled the end of women's willingness to submit themselves to the silliness of fashion – but of course it didn't. When the high street stores tell us that we should raise our hemlines or wear flared trousers, we end up having to – because pretty soon they don't sell anything else, and we can't bear to look too different from our contemporaries. It's the same with our bodies.

In the 1960s Twiggy came along with her flat chest and knock knees, and suddenly we all wanted to look like that, even though our body structures and builds are entirely different. Now we are told that Dianne Brill is the figure of the 90s. That's all very well for those who are 1.8 m (6′) tall with 40–23–40 (100–57–100 cm) figures. But what about the rest of us? Do we, like those before us, upset ourselves because we keep on failing to change? Or do we try to like ourselves the way we are?

Guilty secrets: culpability and the dieting obsession

Each culture has developed its own ideals of physical beauty. In some societies, it is almost as problematic to be thin as it is for us to be fat in our western world. In the West, the pressures on both men and women to conform to a rather slender ideal have given birth to a new national sport: dieting.

We have already mentioned Terence's reference to the Roman mothers who starved their daughters prior to marriage, to make them desirable. This is not the only reference to early dieting habits. The physician and surgeon Galen considered 'excessive corpulency' to be a disease, and the great Hippocrates was most insistent: 'Those who are uncommonly fat die more quickly than the lean.' A glance at those athletic young men and women chasing each other around Grecian urns is enough to make us wonder what life must have been like for an overweight ancient Greek.

Various bizarre ancient therapies have come down to us, including taking exercise before meals, sleep deprivation and rubbing the body with sand (which apparently made it harder and more sleek). By the fourteenth century the Queen of France was advocating sweating rooms – a development which led on to the mid-seventeenth-century fashion for sweating, bleeding and purging. Already people were happy to damage their health in order to become thin. Only too often they damaged their health and stayed fat.

The great dieting debate gained momentum in the nineteenth century, as stern morality and self-discipline became the order of the day. The death of the legendary Daniel Lambert (who weighed over 330 kg, 52 stone) at the age of 40 in 1809 provoked a series of pamphlets on the evils of obesity.

William Wadd's *Cursory Remarks on Corpulence* (1816) was one of the first papers to talk of obesity as a disease, with discernible causes (inactivity, luxurious living and heredity) and treatments (a vegetarian diet, exercise and regular medicinal draughts of vinegar). He agreed, along with many others, that fatness and stupidity were inextricably linked – a fallacy that has persisted in western popular thought right up to the present day. A notable feature of Wadd's paper is a reference to a certain Dr Fleming's famous treatment for corpulence. The unfortunate sufferer was forced to drink one ounce of Castile soap, dissolved in milk or water, three times a day.

The debate reached a peak in the 1860s, with the publication of a paper by one William Banting, a London undertaker. Banting had succeeded in losing 20 kg (46 lbs) through a high-protein, low-carbohydrate diet which doctors now condemn as horribly unhealthy. At the time it caused such a sensation that the word 'banting' (meaning dieting) passed into the language.

A spate of other medical papers appeared, advocating a variety of dietary remedies ranging from vinegar of squills, raw beefsteak and hot water, to smoking all day long and drinking claret. There is no record of whether any of them worked, but it seems pretty unlikely.

The following advertisement, published in *Advice to Stout People* (1883), illustrates the way in which the dieting industry began to grow in the later nineteenth century:

TO STOUT PEOPLE

FIFTY DOZEN GENUINE
JOHANNESBURG SCHLOSSAGE
VINTAGE 1868

at 96s per dozen, in their original cases, landed May, 1873

This wine is particularly recommended to Stout People by the most eminent Physicians; it takes out the watery substance from the fat and puts sinew in its place; gives strength to the body, long life and health; and what it does to the body, so it acts upon the mind, giving fresh nerve by its creating power.

HENRY DE LASPEE, 86 & 87 FLEET ST EC 4

Attitudes towards fat became more critical as the century wore on. The public were told that excess body weight was unhealthy, burdensome, unattractive, and the cause of every possible misfortune: mental retardation, sterility, hysteria, respiratory disease and sudden death (to name but a few). Wadd had already drawn his readers' attention to 'their susceptibility to contagion, and according to some accounts, their danger of combustion'. Readers of the 'Medicus' column in the *Girl's Own Paper* for 12 November 1892, were informed (p. 103) that: 'a fat child can never be a clever one, although he may be, and generally is, a precious disagreeable one to all but his parents'. For the first time, large people were really made to feel that they could not live worthwhile lives unless they became thinner.

Worst of all, according to the 'experts', corpulence was curable and therefore being large was a moral fault. Obesity was supposedly caused by gluttony, which was therefore a form of self-abuse. The anonymous author of *Advice to Stout People* (pp. 15–16) puts the point of view in a particularly unpleasant way:

I would in fact make obesity penal, as calling for special legislation whereby the police would be justified in arresting oleaginous pedestrians, clapping them onto the scales at the nearest police station and if they exceeded a certain number of feet in circumference or weight, at once procure their summary imprisonment, without the option of a fine. The streets would be cleared of these fleshy obstructions; besides which, if the Law recognizes attempted suicide as a crime in one way, why not in another?

Strangely enough, while all this scaremongering was going on, the 'experts' still agreed that the ideal female form was not thin. Perfection was 'embonpoint' – an appealing degree of plumpness.

A confusing state of affairs, which must have left many women wondering just exactly what society *did* want them to look like.

42

Daring to be different

The message of this book is that being large is neither good nor bad – any more than being thin is.

The message of this chapter is that there are almost as many different and conflicting attitudes towards large people as there are cultures and years in the history of the world. In every age and in every country there have been people who were made to feel that they were somehow wrong – simply because they differed from the accepted norm.

The other message is that many attitudes across the years have been foolish, misguided, even dangerous. We now know that many of the old 'remedies' are harmful to health, and there is no reason to think that we have all the answers even now. Drinking soap or swallowing a tapeworm is just as likely to kill you as it is to make you lose weight. Today's revolutionary new diet may well be tomorrow's standing joke.

The answer is not to say that fat is good and thin is bad: that is just another form of discrimination. We need acceptance – by others, and of ourselves. There is no such thing as perfection, but beauty is a commodity that is not limited to thin people. We can all have a share in it. We are not here to be pitied or to feel bad about ourselves. We are here to respect ourselves, to live ordinary lives and to stop denying ourselves the things we want, simply because we're afraid that others might think we're not perfect.

Accept that your body image is a product of cultural and historical influences, and not an objective judgement. Then you can set about judging yourself less harshly.

Further reading

Rethinking Obesity, Paul Ernsberger PhD and Paul Haskew, available from: Human Sciences Press, 72 5th Avenue, New York NY 10011-8004, USA Tel: 212 243 6000

Girth Control, Henry T. Finck (New York: Harper and Row, 1923)

Obesity in Egypt, G. Sobhy (Cairo: Faculty of Medicine, 1928)

The Roseto Story, J. G. Bruhn and S. Wolf (University of Oklahoma Press). This study is quoted in *Radiance*, Winter 1988, p. 42.

3

In Our Image:
Women, the Media and the Arts

Are large women a special case? Organizations like the London Fat Women's Group would argue that they are. A cursory glance at the tabloid press is sufficient to reveal a persistent obsession with the shape and size of women's bodies.

Images of slenderness are all around us. Dieting is an international obsession; and day after day TV and magazines bring us pictures of thin women enjoying themselves, thin women achieving their dreams and thin women winning the love of thin and handsome men. The message is clear: being a thin woman is good, powerful and sexy.

But what about images of largeness? How are big women portrayed, and why? Do the images we see merely reflect current attitudes, or can they also influence and even alter them? If so, then maybe there is some light at the end of the tunnel.

A figure of fun?

According to one American author, 'A fat man is a joke, and a fat woman is two jokes – one on herself and one on her husband' (quoted in *Why Be Fat?* by Dr Cecil Webb-Johnson). Humour, as you might say, is a funny thing and it has seized upon the stereotypical fat lady with an almost insane glee.

Seaside postcards, mother-in-law jokes, jokes about old maids, feminists and lesbians – they are all variations on the 'fat lady' theme. The viewer or listener takes it for granted that 'fat' also means lazy, ugly, greedy, overbearing, stupid and undesirable. If a man is foolish enough to marry a big woman, then he must be sexually inadequate, submissive, and equally stupid and undesirable. Take the following examples of seaside postcards:

- picture of small car driving along with two occupants: the driver (a small, balding man with protuberant ears whose hat is too small and who is sweating profusely) and his wife (a huge woman in dowdy clothes; she is shouting angrily at him from the front passenger seat). A sign on the back of the car reads 'Caution: left hand drive'.
- Castle museum: large wife and small husband. Guide (holding axe): 'Have you ever seen an old battleaxe before?' Husband:

'Seen one! Blimey, I've lived with one for the last 30 years!' Onlookers are laughing at the man and his wife.

Humour is about stereotypes and a feeling of superiority. When you laugh at the inept Keystone Cops or the silent movie actor who slips on a banana skin, you are saying: 'I am not like that. I am cleverer. But I am also slightly afraid of the same thing happening to me, so I am laughing to distance myself from the event.'

It's the same with the traditional reaction to large women. Big people do not fit in with the social norm. Unlike the alcoholic, their supposed 'vice' (greed) is there for all to see. Like black people and those with big noses, they are easy targets. There is also the old fear of the power of a big woman, symbolized in her refusal to submit by limiting her size. Postcard artists like Fitzpatrick and Taylor make sure that her exaggerated sexual characteristics cannot be seen as alluring by giving her dowdy clothes, ragged hair, bags under her eyes, a big red nose and a pendulous lower lip.

The recent crop of new 'alternative' comics like *Viz*, *Brain Damage*, *Gas* and *Smut* has enraged more than a few large women. It seems that the less genuinely funny the comic is, the more use is made of gratuitous anti-fat (and anti-woman) jokes. *Ziggy* and the appropriately named *Smut* are arguably the most offensive to date in their treatment of fat women, and *Smut* also parodies fat men in its 'Fat Idle Bastard' strip.

Perhaps most controversy has surrounded *Viz* characters the 'Fat Slags'. So much interest have they generated that they even provoked an article in the *Guardian* ('Comic Strippers', 7 November 1989) and one (Sandra) has appeared in an advertising campaign for Tennent's lager. Sandra and Tracey are promiscuous, greedy, unintelligent and ultimately ridiculous. Yet they are not victims. If they are used, they are also users. Kate Murphy, who wrote the lager advertising campaign, believes: 'They are formidable. They're like Vikings. We wanted somebody people would be scared of. . . . We have nothing to do with jibes about fat ladies.'

The Fat Slags may indeed be formidable. They may even be tragicomic. But Kate Murphy's assertion rings hollow for two reasons. First, is it not a 'jibe' to imply that fat ladies are something to be scared of? And second, if Sandra and Tracey were not fat they would not be regarded as funny – because they would not be stereotypes any more. The 'humour' arises because they mistakenly believe they are 'lush', gorgeous and sexy and because of that behave as though they were. The reader, of course, knows that they are fat

. . . and therefore ugly. It is a pity that a magazine with genuine talent and originality should choose to take this particular well-worn road to instant laughs.

One woman who has become associated with body size and humour is actress Bella Emberg. Bella has worked solely in comedy for the last eight years, but insists:

> I am an actress – I'm not a comedienne. I'm a character actress who – I hope – makes people laugh. I played my first comedy role 25 years ago, on a Stanley Baxter show, and I loved it. If I had to choose one type of work, it would be comedy. I believe it's the hardest thing on this earth. If you've had a dreadful day at the office and you go to see a comedy show, it's very hard for someone like me or like Russ (Abbot) to make you laugh.

Bella has not always been happy with her size: when she was in her mid-twenties she tried to diet and made herself very ill. She recalls: 'My father, who was a big man, said to me, "Look – you're meant to be large. You're going to be large, so live with it." And I have ever since.'

Indeed, if she had not been large, Bella would never have met up with Russ Abbot and created the now-famous figure of Blunderwoman. How does she react to those people who criticize her work as demeaning to fat women?

> I love Blunderwoman very much. She's a truly funny character. She's simple, of course – I mean, she's so dim, but it doesn't matter because the character of Cooperman is equally dim. . . . Occasionally I do meet people who think I *am* Blunderwoman. But they don't treat me as if I'm stupid. Fat ladies have come up to me and said 'Thank you for what you're doing'. Fat ladies have a heart and soul like anybody else.

It hasn't been laughter all the way for Bella Emberg. There have been times when remarks about her size have really hurt her. She remembers:

> I did 'Save the Children' with Russ and a reader's letter in the *Sun* or the *Star* said they'd never seen such a fat, ugly woman. And that hurt. A couple of years ago there was an article in one of the tabloids on the 'largest and most revolting' man and woman. The man was Cyril Smith and I 'won' the ladies' title. I thought 'I know I'm not everybody's cup of tea', but it really did hurt.

On the other hand, there have been magical moments too. Miss Emberg was once playing a fairy in pantomime: 'I had to sing "Nobody loves a fairy when she's 40", and then disappear into the darkness. One night I sang it and as the lights went down, a little voice rang out from the audience: "But I do".'

Making fun of large women can be cheap and all too easy. Actress Annette Badland vividly recalls her one and only appearance on 'The Dick Emery show':

It was years ago. If I could have been bigger and older, they would have liked it even better. Dick Emery was sitting on a park bench, with his transistor radio beside him. I was just employed to walk on, sit on his transistor radio and squash it, and walk away. I thought after that, 'I'm not doing that again – it really has no wit.' I do have a sense of humour about myself. I do a lot of comedy and I know that's often because I'm big, but I won't do things that I know are simply ridiculing my size.

Attitudes are so deeply entrenched that it really takes no talent to encourage people to ridicule someone's body size. Where talent does come in is in creating an 'alternative' humour which invites the audience to identify with the large woman – share her experiences and laugh with her. It is this striving for identification rather than alienation which has made comediennes like Victoria Wood and Dawn French the heroines of large women everywhere.

French and Saunders work hard to avoid predictable, facile 'fatist' humour – as does Victoria Wood. Although Ms Wood is not as large as she once was, she continues to appeal to large women because she shows 'ordinary' women winning the day in the face of thinner or more glamorous opposition.

The message that humour should portray is that body size is irrelevant in terms of success, attractiveness, self-esteem. That, big or small, it's how you see yourself that counts. Comedy series like 'Roseanne' show that it can be done. If you put yourself down, the world will be quick to follow suit. Putting things off because of your size is like living your life in suspended animation – and every one of us deserves better than that.

Picture this . . . the visual image of large women

A visual image has enormous power to reinforce or to alter accepted attitudes. But how many positive images of large women do we see around us?

An awareness of the situation has prompted Barbara Shores and Diana Pollard, co-founders of Rotunda Press, to plan a positive photographic record of fat women. Barbara hopes to gather together pictures of fat women from birth to adulthood, capturing their development and their beauty in a photographic record. You too can prepare a file of positive images – not only pictures of yourself, but of other people: famous large people, large beauties, people you admire and so on. Pictures of other members of your family will help you to see how you fit into the scheme of things.

Learning to appreciate what is good about the way you look is an important part of accepting your size. Too many large people – especially women – dismiss any representation of a large person as 'ugly' or 'disgusting', and accustoming yourself to positive images is one way to help yourself acquire a whole new set of values.

Scientific studies have shown that attitudes are passed on very early in life. Even very young children respond negatively to pictures of large people. In 'The Goddess is Fat' in the collection *Shadow on a Tightrope*, 'Kelly' explains:

> One of these studies was done in Manhattan. Eight groups of children were asked to rate seven photos of other children, as to who they would most want to be friends with, and who they would least want to be friends with. Seven of the eight groups put the fat child last. . . . The report . . . didn't describe all of the other photos. Only five of the seven photos were described: one child pictured was in a wheelchair, one was a child missing an arm, one was 'normal', one had a facial disfigurement, and one was fat. The one group of children that did not rate the fat child last was a group of working-class Jewish children. They rated the fat child third.

In a poll of students, respondents were asked to assign adjectives to two pictures: one of a fat child and one of a thin child. The thin child was described as 'trustworthy, would make a good friend, nice, fun, easy to get along with, smart, happy'. The fat child provoked the response 'dirty, liar, mean, lazy, tends to get into fights, ugly, stupid'. Two-year-old children were given a choice between a fat rag doll and a thin one, and most preferred the thin one. By the age of ten, 100 per cent of them opted for the thin doll.

In the light of these results, it is obvious that it will be an uphill struggle to readjust the image of the large person. Parents influence their children from birth, so it is at parents that we must direct positive visual images.

If we look at art through the ages, the overwhelming impression is one of slenderness. Of course, there is the work of Rubens, Titian, Correggio and Renoir, full of relaxed and smiling women who would never dream of apologizing for not being a size 10. On the other hand, these pictures are very much islands in a sea of slenderness. After all, until a century or so ago largeness was far less common because of poor nutrition. If you were big, you were lucky: you would probably survive.

Today's western abundance of food has given prestige to thinness, and it seems likely that that prestige will continue to grow as nutritionists urge us to embrace a New Age diet and lifestyle. New Age men and women, they claim, will be very different from the bulky people who have emerged since the development of intensive farming techniques boosted our food supplies in the nineteenth century.

The new ideal of feminine beauty will be anything but voluptuous. Fed on an organic and semi-vegetarian diet, she will be short in stature with a boyish (some would say bony) figure. Unfortunately, this sort of talk merely emphasizes the old prejudice against fat women: 'Ah well, she's only fat because she eats chips and cream cakes all day long.'

All is not lost, however. Beryl Cook continues to bring us wonderful, humorous, affectionate glimpses of a more realistic world in which men and women love their bodies – bulges, wrinkles and all. There are pictures of statuesque women in sexy underwear, rolypoly strippers, stockbrokers' and vicars' wives sitting, naked except for their hats, around a tea-table eating cucumber sandwiches.

Perhaps the most powerful visual image is that provided by advertisers and the fashion industry. In America, manufacturers are less apprehensive about using 'queen-sized' models in their fashion advertising. So you might open a magazine to find a Triumph advertisement featuring a large, smiling, unselfconscious model in her underwear – or a thoroughly glamorous size 24 modelling luxury evening tights.

The British magazines *Extra Special* and *Cachet* tried to create an atmosphere in which this type of visual glamour could thrive – but sadly, both magazines had a relatively brief lifespan. Lingerie manufacturers in this country insist that customers want advertisements to be 'aspirational' rather than realistic – showing what a woman would like to look like, rather than what she actually *does* look like. Yet women repeatedly say that they want to see images of large people doing ordinary things, leading ordinary lives and looking good. The United States, with its bigger potential market, manages to sustain two magazines for large women (*Big Beautiful Woman* and *Radiance*) and *Magna*, a magazine for big and tall men.

There are then moves to improve the visual image of large women. London fashion shop Big Clothes has, for example, started a newsletter which includes photographs of big women dressed up and looking beautiful. And Carol Crawford has set up a new model agency (CJ's) in South London, aimed at training big men and women to feel and present themselves in a glamorous way. She is particularly irritated by fashion catalogues which display 'outsize' clothes on slim models – giving large customers the impression that they are not thought presentable enough to model their own clothes. Carol recently staged her first sponsored fashion show, and looks forward to future events.

Carol (a size 16) explains:

> My aim is to give confidence and a sense of importance to large people as we have to live with our size. A large person can portray glamour and beauty just as well as anyone else and I think we should be given the opportunity to express ourselves in that way.

Up in lights

Stage and screen are tough worlds for large women. Look at the way in which Elizabeth Taylor has been hounded every time she has the effrontery to put on a bit of weight. 'She's still a great actress,' her showbiz friends assure us – as though the size or shape of her body had a bearing on her ability to act.

Are there 'fat' parts and 'thin' parts – two worlds that must never meet, let alone overlap? Is the fat actress doomed to play the schoolmarm while the thin girl gets all the romantic leads? Is it impossible to read the news competently unless you are thin?

Television and films demand a particularly close visual link between actors and the parts they play. There are many cases of actors and actresses having to lose or put on huge amounts of weight just for one part – and then transform their bodies into a completely different shape for the next job. Bob Hoskins, for example, had to lose 9 kg (20 lbs) in two weeks for his role in the film 'Heart Condition' – hardly a very healthy rate at which to lose weight. Meryl Streep had to put on 13 kg (30 lbs) for her role as 'dingo baby' mother Lindy Chamberlain, and then lose it all again. To quote an article in the *Sunday Express Magazine* (27 August 1989): 'Doctors agree that when actors undergo dramatic weight changes, the only thing likely to be healthier at the end of it is their bank balance.'

There is tremendous pressure on actors and actresses to be a particular shape – to use their bodies as a tool to get work. Lynn Redgrave achieved fame in the 1960s with *Georgy Girl*, but:

> I knew that unless I lost weight I was going to be absolutely stuck in a niche, playing someone who was jolly and ungainly. I felt I could play many more people but when I saw the film I realized that anybody looking at me wasn't going to know that. It was all very well thinking I had all these Juliets inside me, but there was no way people were going to say, 'Take that girl and put her opposite Romeo'.

So she set about becoming 'professionally thin' and was caught for years in the vicious circle of bingeing and starving.

One woman who has challenged the established film world is German actress Marianne Sägebrecht – another heroine for many large women. The success of her warm, humorous and sexy roles in films like *Sugar Baby* and *Baghdad Café* have forced casting directors to think about casting their net wider.

Nevertheless, in view of all the pressures on actresses, it is a brave woman who decides to stop fighting her body and work with it the way it is. Actresses Annette Badland and Caroline Ryder have done just that.

Caroline's story

It never really occurred to Caroline Ryder that she might not be able to become an actress because she was too fat. It's just as well that she didn't decide against trying, because she would have missed out on a successful television career which has already included parts in the series 'Truckers' and, more recently, 'Chelworth'.

It wasn't until she got to drama school that Caroline realized the pressures that would be on her to change her appearance and fit in with the traditional image of the slender, glamorous actress:

> Previously I'd been in a boarding school atmosphere, and nobody would have been so impolite as to say 'look – you're too fat'. I was very taken aback when it was pointed out to me, but even then I was a bit obstinate.
>
> I did slim down quite a lot and then I went to London. I wasn't very happy, and put on a fair amount of weight. All they said was 'lose weight, lose weight'. I remember on the day I left, the Principal said 'You've never really listened to a word I said, have

you?' I said 'No, not really'. And she said 'Well, you'll be all right'.

Despite all the advice to change her appearance, young Caroline was not easily swayed. She felt she had the potential to make it in the profession just as she was:

> I looked at myself and thought, 'This is the shape and size I am. Am I going to fight it or be happy like I am now?' I thought 'How many people in this life are actually thin anyway?' So I decided I would promote myself as someone who *isn't* glamorous or thin; someone who's willing to say 'Yes – I'm not your average pint-sized actress'. My marketability is quite different from that of most young actresses.

The gamble has paid off. In fact, Caroline has found her 80 kg (12½ stone), size 14–16 figure a great help in starting her off as an actress:

> I've worked on average more than the majority of my drama school year. . . . I wanted to maintain my individuality, and it's worked. I'm very marketable, according to my agent. I've got something slightly different to offer, and I'm willing to admit it. One actress I know is also large but she won't admit it even to herself, so she doesn't go up for the parts. It's a vicious circle.

One possible drawback of being a larger-than-average actress is the more limited range of parts available. Caroline feels that this is partly due to prejudice on the part of writers. She was delighted when she landed the role of Dibs in 'Chelworth', and hopes that it will open up new horizons for her:

> I won't get cast as the Titanias of this world, but I would like to play some more romantic parts. Take a character like Jane Eyre: how do we know she wasn't a bit tubby? She was certainly plain. There's no good reason why I couldn't play the part, but I doubt if I would ever be cast.

Annette's story
Annette Badland is a size 20–24. A well-respected and versatile actress, she is perhaps still best known for her role as the original secretary in 'Bergerac'.

Like Caroline, Annette had no intention of letting her size stop her from becoming an actress. At East 15 drama school, she was given the opportunity to play the full range of leading roles, irrespective of size: 'they gave me a lot of things to do that now I'm out in the profession I wouldn't get – Titania, Norah in *A Doll's House*, and so on.' This hardly prepared her for the big bad world of professional acting, in which even radio parts are cast from *Spotlight* – a photographic directory. So even in the invisible medium of radio it looks as if Annette will never be a Juliet.

Yet Annette is very satisfied with the direction of her career:

I've been lucky and have done a whole range of things. I haven't been blocked into sitcoms. I work a lot. On the other hand, TV is about image and often very immediate image, so they don't tend to take risks. They just go for the external picture and that's it.

'Bergerac' gave Annette her first big break on television, playing the part of the detective's secretary at the Bureau des Etrangers. In fact, this was one example of a casting risk:

Robert Banks Stewart, who created the series, felt he took an enormous risk casting me in the first place – he thought it was very adventurous. I was quite pleased with the part, especially when I was given a boyfriend (Richard Griffiths) who was a mountaineer –though I was disappointed at the decision to make him big, too.

Annette emphasizes the powerful effect of showing positive images of big women on prime-time television:

Public response was amazing. Men were saying 'This is great. Can I have your address and can I mend your car?' Women were saying 'It's just smashing having someone on TV that I can relate to.' Advertising says that people want to see the very best, the image they want to be themselves, and not reality. But I don't think that's particularly true – not from the letters I received.

Although Annette admits that she would quite like to 'try being thin', she suspects that her work would dry up. On one occasion she did lose 19 kg (3 stone) and found reactions towards her changing – not always for the better. She is happy with her size nowadays, and grateful for the opportunities which it has opened up:

I have a much better time than many of my contemporaries, who sit at home for eleven months of the year, because I'm something specific. I do work a lot – though the competition is greater nowadays. When I started, I didn't fit into a slot. I was too young. If I'd been uglier, that might have been all right, because fat and ugly was a concept that TV companies could handle. You had to be old and a harridan or a slob. To be young and fat – no. I think things like 'Bergerac' must have changed things slightly.

Even now, Annette feels that the range of parts is too limited. A director has expressed interest in casting her in a love story, and she very much hopes that the project will work out. But she regrets the fact that:

I know there are things that I should be seen for because of my emotional ability, talent and age range, but which I will never be considered for. They would never consider a fat person as a career woman, or a lover, or a wife. It's assumed that the bigger you become, the less intelligent, the less sexual, the less emotionally sensitive you are – which is ridiculous.

Newsreaders and television discrimination

It is not only in acting that size has a bearing on success. When was the last time you saw a fat newsreader or TV presenter? When Terry Wogan complains about his weight, it just makes those of us who really are big feel worse about ourselves. At the other end of the scale is Selina Scott, telling the world 'I want to be fatter but I can't put on weight' (*Today*, 22 December 1989).

There really is discrimination against large people – especially women – on television. Shelley Bovey (author of *Being Fat is not a Sin*) is an experienced broadcaster but has never made it onto the screen, simply because of her size. Gabrielle, a large woman and a television researcher, used to work on the game show 'Blankety Blank'. She recalls:

Producers on quiz shows didn't want fat people on their programmes. One really ticked me off once for putting a fat woman on a show. He called her 'fat and ugly'. I think a lot of men equate fat with ugliness and being a slob. I had an idea for a magazine programme called 'Fat Chat', but couldn't raise enough interest in the project.

The pop world

In the world of pop music, things are not much different. Barry White and Demis Roussos may be able to forge thriving careers as sex symbols, but a large woman has to have a truly exceptional voice before anyone will take her seriously. The extremely beautiful and talented Alison Moyet is one who has succeeded in spite of her size. Unfortunately she seems uncomfortable with her body and cloaks it in black, only paying attention to her face which is always immaculately made-up. Some singers, like Gloria Estefan, take the line of least resistance and lose weight in order to boost their careers through sex appeal. Moving in the same world as Estefan, singer Chaka Khan has faced nothing but ridicule since she put on weight – though musically it makes not the slightest difference to her performance. Even in the world of opera, the substantial silhouettes of Montserrat Caballe and Joan Sutherland are beginning to give way to the comparative slenderness of Kiri Te Kanawa. When will it end? Perhaps with the growth in popularity of African and Afro-Caribbean music, whose singers are so often big and beautiful.

Words, words, words: the written image

In a highly literate society like ours, it is hardly surprising that words are so influential. Reputations and opinions can be made or lost on the strength of a single article in a Sunday tabloid. Everywhere there are people trying to write novels, poems or song lyrics. It is impossible not to be influenced.

A poet's eye view

The most remarkable insights – and the most positive images – are to be found in poetry. All of the hurt, the prejudice, the voluptuousness and the consolations of being large can be found in verse.

We all learned at school those famous lines by Frances Cornford:

> O fat white woman whom nobody loves,
> Why do you walk through the fields in gloves. . . ?

So being a fat white woman makes you inherently unlovable? G. K. Chesterton disagreed. In fact, he even wrote a reply – *The Fat White Woman Speaks* – in which the much-maligned fat woman informs the poet that her devoted husband is waiting for her at the end of the field! The trials and tribulations of being labelled as 'fat' have inspired a good deal of modern feminist poetry – some amusing, some despairing, some defiant. In Maureen Burge's *The Diet*, a woman sits in a pub tormented by the sight of people enjoying themselves: she's on a diet.

In the end, visions of crisps and chicken and chips are too much to bear and she rebels:

> No I can't keep quiet
> I'll shout, Bugger the diet
> I'm absolutely starving

Canadian poet Christine Donald specializes in writing about the inner pain of being fat, and in challenging society's assumptions about large women. Take her *Poor Old Fat Woman*, for example:

> Poor old fat woman, whither bound?
> Home to my hearth, kind sir, she said.
> Poor old fat woman, living alone!
> I live with a woman who loves me, she said.
> Poor old fat woman, lonely and tired!
> We've plans for this evening, sir, she said.
> No husband for you, poor old fat woman, eh!
> I've never wanted one, sir, she said.
> Poor old fat woman, what do you want?
> Nothing that you can give, sir, she said,
>   And you're wasting your time
>   And you're wasting mine
> So push off and do something useful instead.

Ms Donald talks about thin women who think they're fat, thin lovers of fat people who wonder if they should accept them as they are or persuade them to diet, and the many insecurities of being large.

If Christine Donald is the poet of anguish and rebellion, Grace Nichols is the poet of positivity. She has created a wonderful character – the 'fat black woman' who embodies all the most joyful, humorous and positive qualities of being a large woman.

The fat black woman is a product of her culture – proud of her body and its fertile sensuality, powerful and witty – but lives in a western society that refuses to cater for her type of abundant beauty. In *The Fat Black Woman Goes Shopping*:

> Nothing soft and bright and billowing
> to flow like breezy sunlight
> when she walking . . .
> . . . the choice is lean
>
> Nothing much beyond size 14.

But she remains undeterred. She has no doubt that big is beautiful, natural, useful:

> Fat is a dream
> in times of lean
>> fat is a darling
>> a dumpling
>> a squeeze
>> fat is cuddles
>> up a baby's sleeve
>> and fat speaks for itself. (*A Fat Poem*)

Speaking for herself, the fat black woman refuses to compromise her own self-image simply to fit in with the way her lovers might expect her to look. In *The Invitation*, she explains that if her weight had been too much for her, she would have dieted – but as it is she sees no need to change. She feels fine – 'target-light' – and full of promise, so she issues this invitation to her lover:

> Come up and see me sometime
> My breasts are huge exciting
> amnions of watermelon
>> your hands can't cup
> my thighs are twin seals
>> fat slick pups . . .

A man's view is provided by Jamaican poet James Berry, who describes his poem *Boonoonoonoos Gal* as being 'in praise of the larger woman – the round, big-bosomed, big-bottomed lady. Boonoonoonoos is a Jamaican word with an African sound.'

Between them, modern poets are challenging the old prejudices and assumptions about large women. Grace Nichols's 'fat black woman' and James Berry's 'Boonoonoonoos gal' are sisters to the smiling women of Rubens and Renoir.

In the news

We may be big – but are we news? The tabloid obsession with diets, plastic surgery and 'ballooning' celebrities is enough to convince any visiting Martian that the only important factor in our society is body size. If we're not careful, it might convince us too.

A right royal furore

There cannot be many people in this country who are not aware of the fluctuations in the Duchess of York's waistline. The tabloid press have kept us posted with monotonous regularity, whether we liked it or not.

Viewed objectively, Sarah has never been particularly large. More to the point, even if she had been enormous, would that have been news? Presumably she could open hospitals and make speeches just as competently whatever size she was. But it's all a question of image.

Royal girth has always provoked a certain amount of comment (George IV and Edward VII inspired some vicious cartoons) but never before have members of the Royal Family been so visible, so accessible and so much like Hollywood film stars. The press expects them to be physically perfect, according to a set of very stringent specifications. Even the unfortunate Prince Edward's premature baldness has produced a few critical comments. The fact is that if the Royals – and the ladies in particular – fail to fit the image the tabloids want to project, then the tabloids will set about getting the message across. It doesn't matter what the readers think: the newspapers shape their opinions, too.

During and after her pregnancy, the Duchess of York was presented to readers as fat, frumpish and unpleasant. As her body became larger, the comments became more and more critical and her personality was described as selfish, bossy, greedy, etc. But by November 1988, she had lost a lot of weight – and the press changed tack once again, the implication being that Fergie now deserved praise because of her self-discipline and determination. The real 'story' – her speech in support of the arts – was relegated to a single brief paragraph.

By January 1989, the Duchess's 'dedication' to losing weight had sparked off a boom in Callanetics – a type of exercise regime designed by Callan Pinckney. The *Sun*'s article: 'How I got flabby Fergie back into shape again: fitness girl's mission' had women flocking to buy Ms Pinckney's book. When, in March, the Duchess admitted to reporters that she had to live on 'fruit . . . raw vegetables (and) just a little protein', no-one sympathized with her – doomed by other people's expectations to live on a boring diet for the rest of her life.

Having succeeded in pressurizing the Duchess into losing weight and dressing as they wished her to, the tabloid press were rather lost for something to complain about. Their next golden opportunity came in January 1990, when the Duchess was pregnant with her second child. Obviously feeling that she had to retain her slender figure, the Duchess ate carefully and put on little weight. 'Ain't she thin!' screeched the *Daily Mirror* (5 January 1990). Not content with forcing the poor woman to diet, the tabloids now criticized her for looking 'gaunt', and hinted that she might be endangering the health of her baby by . . . not eating enough. Each story was accompanied by an unflattering photograph of the Duchess – fleshless face, staring eyes – designed to inspire panic in readers. Perhaps you *can* be too rich and too thin?

Big names?

The manipulation and victimization of the famous does not stop with the Royal Family. Any woman who is in the public eye is scrutinized for potential storylines, and body size is one of the most popular 'angles' of all. Famous people are expected to be 'perfect' people, so they are ruthlessly punished if they do not come up to scratch. Liz Taylor, Chaka Khan, Gloria Estefan, Pam St Clement, Cheryl Baker, Victoria Wood, Barbara Bush . . . the list of women who have provided targets for fat-obsessed journalists is endless.

No news means fat news

If there is no real news around, you can guarantee that the newspapers will be full of trivia about the Martians landing in Wakefield, maneating goldfish . . . and fat ladies. It's not just the *Sunday Sport* with its 'gargantuan gutbuckets' – all the tabloids play the sizism game to some degree.

No-one is immune. Andy Warhol once said that in future we would all be famous for fifteen minutes. If so, the first question every woman will be asked by the reporters is 'what size are you?'. Look at all the stories featuring women. How are they described? The chances are you will find phrases like 'buxom barmaid Cindy', 'voluptous Vera', 'sad blob Natalie', 'plump pedestrian Sandra' and so on. As a rule, the size of the lady has no relevance to the story. Whether you are run over by a bus, mugged or awarded a prize, they will still want to know how much you weigh. If the story really is related to your size (for example, if you have been sacked because you were 'too large') the tabloids will be even more delighted to make fun of you.

It is perfectly possible to report a size-related story without being salacious. It just doesn't happen very often. Take the example of the 'fat hotel'. American comedian and nutritionist Dick Gregory set up a weight loss programme for very large people and hired a hotel. His 'guests' were thirteen people who needed to lose a lot of weight for health reasons. The story was reported by both the *News of the World* and the *Independent*. In 'What it means to be big in America', the *Independent* reported the facts and gave a few biographical details of the people involved. Fair enough. But the tabloid version – 'Diet or Die!' is yet another example of the way in which a perfectly ordinary story can be milked for the sensational, the grotesque and the tasteless.

The *Independent* reporter (Sue Woodman) talks dispassionately of 'overweight', 'obese people' and 'weight loss programmes'. The *News of the World* wallows in such phrases as 'porky pals', 'desperate fatties', 'mammoth men and women' and 'blankets of blubber' and implies that all the people on the programme are fighting an inevitable death sentence. It also includes voyeuristic pictures of fat people exercising.

Quite apart from the question of journalistic style is the fundamental question: is it news? Why do the press assume that people will be interested in subjects which so many of us find either insensitive or irrelevant? If we don't say anything, how will they know what we think?

A change for the better?

People who write have the power to change the way in which other people perceive the world. Accurate and sensitive writing by and about large people can help other people to empathize. And by changing what is written about large people, by projecting a more positive image, there is no reason why fundamental prejudices cannot also be changed.

One way to ensure that positive views of fat people are available is to set up your own publishing house, and this is exactly what Barbara Shores (manager of a rock band) and Diana Pollard (a catering consultant) have just done, by launching Rotunda, the first-ever fat women's press in Britain. Their first project is the reissue of the influential American book, *Shadow on a Tightrope*. If that proves successful, there will be more and bigger ventures.

What can I do about it?

Rotunda Press is good news for fat people, especially women; but at the other end of the scale, the tasteless and the sensational can only do harm. If you feel strongly about something in the news or on the television, there are things you can do:

- Write or telephone the journalist involved. Make a noise. Get your family and friends to make a noise too. Think about joining one of the support groups which we talked about in the chapter on attitudes. Concerted action is more likely to be effective, and it is much easier to be brave in the company of others.

- Get together a petition (I know of at least one woman who is organizing one against a notorious tabloid newspaper).
- If you have good ideas, make sure people know about them. Supply ideas for TV programmes which could incorporate positive images of fat people doing ordinary things – without drawing attention to their presence.
- Draw, paint, take photographs, or write articles for the mainstream press – anything that makes people more aware of large people and the problems they face in breaking down stereotypes.

If we don't do anything to help ourselves, no-one is going to do it for us. It is only by action – and not by sitting around feeling indignant or sorry for ourselves – that we can hope to replace some of the negative images with positive ones.

Useful addresses

CJ's Modelling Agency (Carol Crawford)
Flat 4
134 Woodside Green
South Norwood
London SE25 5EW
Tel: 081 655 0441

Ugly Enterprises Ltd (agency specializing in 'ordinary' and unusual models)
Tigress House
256 Edgware Road
London W2 1DS
Tel: 071 402 5564

Further reading

Shadow on a Tightrope, ed. Lisa Schoenfielder and Barb Wieser (originally published in America by Aunt Lute Press; available in the UK from Rotunda Press)
Being Fat is not a Sin, Shelley Bovey (London: Pandora, 1989)
Fat: a Love Story, Barbara Wersba (London: Bodley Head, 1987)
Why Be Fat?, Cecil Webb-Johnson (London: Mills and Boon, 1923)

The Fat Woman's Joke, Fay Weldon (London: Hodder & Stoughton, 1982)

The Fat Black Woman's Poems, Grace Nichols (London: Virago, 1984)

The Fat Woman Measures Up, Christine Donald (Charlottetown, Canada: Ragweed Press, 1987)

Internal Affairs, Jill Tweedie (London: Heinemann, 1986)

4

Big Deal: Fat Men Today

Nobody loves a fat man (American proverb)
Everybody loves a fat man (American proverb)

Thin people tend to assume that, because little is said about large men, they must all lead a carefree existence of beer and skittles. In fact, a glance at the two proverbs quoted above reveals that attitudes to fat men are, and always have been, ambivalent. A fat man can be cast as a strong man or a weakling, a hero or a villain, a mastermind or a dunce. A fat actor can play Othello – and never an eyebrow raised – though Hamlet is tantalizingly out of bounds.

Unlike large women, large men as yet have no fixed role in society. But as the health evidence is stacked up against them, and the fashion industry nags them to wear more fashionable clothes, they are beginning to feel the pressure.

According to Liz Swinden, a member of the London Fat Women's Group, 'It's easier for men, for whom being fat, or big, is often synonymous with being powerful.' But is that really the case nowadays – and was it ever true?

What is a fat man, anyway?

Diana Pollard, of the London Fat Women's Group, divides fat women into two categories: those who are over the statutory size 12, and those who suffer from the '90 kg, 200 lb plus syndrome'. The first group are sneered at and criticized, but it is only the very large women who suffer practical problems of access, seating, mobility etc.

So what about men? Is there a weight or a size at which a man ceases to be a thin man with a paunch and becomes a fat man? If we take clothes as a guide, a man with a waist above 95 cm (38″) faces problems in buying garments off-the-peg. Yet if that man is also tall, he may not be fat. A very short man like actor Danny De Vito is obviously going to look rounder than a tall man with the same girth. There are no absolutes. Fat is as much a subjective judgement of the eye as it is a question of weight or size.

Take athletes, for example. Is a weightlifter fat? Is a heavyweight boxer fat? Is Geoff Capes fat? All of them probably weigh more than they should in terms of actuarial 'height–weight' tables, but their weight consists of muscle, not fat. Wrestlers are another case in point. They are often very large indeed, yet they lead punishing lifestyles and their size is their strength. Gary retired recently after 26 years as professional wrestler 'Catweazle'. He is in no doubt at all that big can also be fit:

> I was in the wrestling business for 26 years. Wrestlers have to do a lot of training and develop their muscles – you go for fitness. In that game you need stamina. It's not just size: you need that stamina and you need to know what you're doing. I'm 2 m (6'3") and weigh 100–120 kg (16½–17 stone).

Of course, the drawback for big sportsmen is that as soon as they stop training their muscles tend to turn to fat. Gary admits

> I've put on a bit of weight since I stopped wrestling, and I've got a belly like Michelin man. I think that as long as you're happy it doesn't matter what size you are – though I do worry sometimes about health.

According to Gary, being big does not necessarily mean being unattractive either. The 'big, strong and macho' image of the wrestler appeals to many women:

> Being a wrestler is a bit like being a pop star. There are all sorts of women – 'ring rats' we call them – who go for wrestlers. Doctors, housewives, the lot. A lot of them like large men – even the villains. They like the aggression, I think, and the manliness. Women who've seen you on television say 'I didn't realize how big you were', and they like that. They expect a wrestler to be big. Look at Giant Haystacks – he's 2.1 m (6'11'), and weighs 200 kg (42 stone).

Not every big man is a happy man. Very large men face practical problems and sometimes discrimination. Men who develop 'feminine' characteristics such as breasts and large bottoms often find themselves the butt of cruel jokes about their virility. But it's clear that 'big' and 'fat' are terms that have no specific definition.

The weight of tradition

Historian Edward Shorter explains that, traditionally, men have always been better nourished than their womenfolk, getting the lion's share in working-class and peasant families. The idea (often misguided) was that 'men's work' required greater energy, so what family resources there were went into producing big, strong, healthy men.

Even today, it is not unusual in a family for the mother to serve herself last and deprive herself of the best food, even though she has prepared the meal. Hers is the smallest portion, too, because she is on a diet yet again – and besides, it isn't 'polite' for a woman to eat as much as a man. This is an ancient tradition, and one which refuses to die.

Despite his preferential treatment at the dinner-table, the fat man who was also poor was a rarity until the mid-nineteenth century, when improved agricultural methods began to provide more and better food to the lower classes. It is difficult to imagine a Stone Age fat man: he would probably have been too slow to catch his dinner! On the other hand, historians have suggested that it is the fatter people generally who were equipped for survival in the Ice Age – so it is those with a greater than average capacity to store surplus energy whose genetic lines have continued to the present day (Anne Scott Beller, *Fat and Thin*, 1980).

Until relatively recent times, a fat man was generally a wealthy man. Whereas women were urged to achieve a degree of 'embonpoint' and no more, in men a well-covered body was often regarded as attractive, healthy and a sign of cheerfulness and prosperity.

There were a few dissenting voices, particularly in the wake of the death in 1809 of Daniel Lambert – at well over 330 kg (52 stone) Britain's fattest man. Eminent surgeons like William Wadd reprimanded British men who tried to emulate this 'prodigy of clogged machinery', and warned them that they were doomed to mental degeneration, immobility and an early grave.

Some men did take notice of what the surgeons said. Indeed, most of the early reducing diets were aimed at men who had had rather too much good living than was good for them. All sorts of arguments were used to persuade men to stop boasting about their weight, and start worrying about it instead. Perhaps one of the most persuasive arguments was the financial one: by the beginning of this century, insurance companies were using height–weight tables and charging an extra premium to anyone they considered too corpulent.

The conflict of traditions is obvious. On the one hand, we have the positive view of fat men as strong, healthy and prosperous – the symbol of plenty and contentment. The view persists that a large appetite is 'greedy' in a woman, but 'healthy' in a man. A fat woman is 'ugly, dirty and lazy', while her much fatter husband is 'a growing boy', 'well setup', 'a big lad' and so on. Restaurants still serve up 'man-sized' portions and expect them to be eaten.

The other traditional view is of the fat man as a monster of uncontrolled appetites – a fat satyr whose appetite for food is matched only by his appetite for depravity. Psychologists have written about a phenomenon they call 'oral rage' or 'alimentary orgasm', describing the almost sexual pleasure which some men derive from gluttony, and their inability to moderate their appetites.

Whether a power-hungry tyrant or a pathetic, weak individual without sexual identity or self-respect, the 'uncontrolled' type of fat man is not judged worthy of respect. Why? Because he *has* no self-respect, no self-control. He is morally degenerate. He is a victim of inflexible Victorian values.

Either way, little consideration is given to the idea that a man might be fat simply because nature intended him to be that way, owing either to a glandular problem or an hereditary predisposition. The fat man – according to tradition – is a man who eats a lot, for whatever reason.

Can't we divorce the man from his fat, view them as two separate identities? Society loves to make judgements about the fat man, but as yet cannot decide whether or not it likes him.

Lean times? What it means to be fat

In a society where thin is beautiful and fat is morally questionable, it is hardly surprising that big men face problems in everyday life. What is surprising is that the 'fat liberation' movement – in Britain at least – has largely ignored them up to now.

What is certain is that a fat man is not always a happy man. He does not always go through life eating cream buns and beaming benignly in the face of the world's taunts and jeers. As early as 1863, William Banting (slimmer extraordinaire and father of the modern dieting obsession) explained that he had lost 46 lb in sheer desperation because he could no longer bear the cruel remarks, the stares and the physical restrictions of being fat.

Banting's diet caught the public imagination, and soon everyone was talking about how terrible it was to be fat. The balance was shifting in favour of stern Victorian values. If a fat man could become a thin man, simply through the exercise of willpower, then he should do so. Only a very weak-willed creature would choose to risk dreadful diseases, ridicule and early death – not to mention the much-publicized danger of spontaneous combustion! Only a man with no sense of responsibility would risk leaving his wife and children without a breadwinner.

Although something of the old 'laugh and grow fat' mentality still exists, the cold draught of Victorian opinion can be felt in insurance offices, doctors' surgeries and health clubs up and down the land. Fat men are beginning to experience similar problems to those of fat women as society demands that individuals conform more and more closely to a given physical stereotype.

Big men today face a whole host of problems, most of which are ignored or dismissed as a joke by the rest of the population. They may include:

- *Discrimination at work*: failing the company medical, being passed over for promotion, being considered incapable of physical effort, lacking authority and losing respect, being considered stupid, greedy and lazy. Many major companies admit that they consider physical fitness and appearance when recruiting at managerial level, and tend to adopt a 'healthy body, healthy mind' approach.
- *Abuse*: insults in the street, jibes about virility and eating habits.
- *Clothes*: the impossibility of buying anything off the peg, or indeed anything fashionable at all – though on the plus side, men's fashions fluctuate less than women's so clothes can be worn for a longer period. The styles are also often more comfortable than those of women's fashions. The recent introduction of the 'Plus' range by Marks and Spencer may herald a move towards more reasonably priced clothes for large men.
- *Practical problems*: everything from the width of cinema seats to the difficulty of getting into a car.
- *Health problems*: research (discussed in Chapter 5) indicates that fat men are more at risk of developing certain diseases (such as heart disease) than fat women. Worrying about your health can also make you ill, particularly if your general practitioner is unsympathetic and makes insensitive comments like 'lose weight or you'll be dead within two years'.
- *Problems with relationships*: although women seem more receptive to large men than men are to large women, relationships can still be a problem. If you feel ashamed or embarrassed about your physical appearance, it can become an ordeal even to put yourself into social situations where you might meet potential partners. Will you be ridiculed or rejected? Will you be ruled out as a sexual partner because of your size?

Andrew is only too aware of the problems of being large. Not only is he a big man in terms of weight (around 110 kg, 18 stone) – he is also 1.9 m (6'5") tall, which makes him a man you simply can't fail to notice.

Even as a child, Andrew was 'on the big side'. He weighed 4.5 kg (9 lb 13 oz) at birth, though he was a month premature! As he says, 'clearly I meant to start as I was going to carry on!'

Everyone in Andrew's family is tall and broad. Even his mother (in her sixties) is 1.7 m (5'8"), and one of his uncles reached an imposing 2 m (6'9"). Andrew takes a size 13 in shoes, and this, added to his fluctuating girth, makes clothing a perennial problem. Even everyday objects like bicycles have to be made to order – at extra cost.

It wasn't until he was fifteen or sixteen that it dawned on Andrew that he was becoming really large. He found he couldn't buy gym clothes or plimsolls, which was a source of great hilarity to his classmates and great embarrassment to him. Suddenly he was bigger and broader than all the adults around him. He felt very unhappy at school, and believes this caused him to be an underachiever: 'Size made me instantly recognizable, so it was hard to be inconspicuous. Hence, any misdemeanours led to retribution that the average little lad might escape.'

The combination of weight and height has brought many problems with it:

> Rules and regulations are very inconsistent. For example, I could join the police if I wanted to, but not the RAF or the submarine service! Physically, I have problems with bus seats and low ceilings etc. . . . Large men are assumed to be big tough guys – policemen, security guards, guardsmen, bouncers etc: a classic example of stereotyping. As such, people tend to assume your intellect is around the level they associate with such 'heavies'. There's also an implicit feeling of violence from 'gorillas' like me!

Andrew now has a successful professional career and is happy in his work. Joining Mensa has strengthened his confidence in his intellectual abilities. Yet he admits that he still lacks confidence in social situations:

> My self-confidence is low, and I do feel that my size has an effect on my personal relationships. However innocently intended, instant comments about size raise self-consciousness and create a negative atmosphere. Parties are awful: all crammed in and too high up to

hear the conversation! I feel accepted at work, so I'm happier with my colleagues and tend to slip away from social contacts.

At the other end of the scale from Andrew is the man who is short and fat. He too can suffer from stereotyping – not as the menacing 'heavy', but as the ever-jolly, rather asexual person who is cast sometimes as the victim and more often than not as the clown. It takes an exceptional strength of personality to break through these preconceived notions and convince others to accept you not as a freak of nature, but as an ordinary human being.

A general lack of sympathy, and pressure from family, friends and workmates to lose weight, can be very demoralizing for any large man. Diana Pollard, of the London Fat Women's Group, explains:

I know a man who's 150 kg (24 stone). He's married to a woman who's about 7 or 8 stone – she's really tiny. His family have taken her aside and said to her that she should deny him sex, threaten to leave him, all kinds of things, to get him to diet. The couple have a young child, and she has been told that she should constantly remind him that he's going to make her a widow and the child an orphan if he 'persists in this obese way of life'.

The thing is, he is a victim of childhood diets. From the age of about seven, his mother looked at him and thought 'You're bigger than all the other boys, so I'd better start doing something about it.' So she put him on a series of diets. From his early childhood, he would go on a diet and lose some weight, then he would be allowed –as a reward – to eat normally. Then his weight would increase beyond what it was before he started the diet. Medical people tell us that this is because the body registers a famine situation and slows down the metabolism.

Diana recognizes the difference that understanding can make to the quality of life for big men. But some people would argue, with the man's family, that if there is a danger to health through being fat, there is a duty to make the man aware of his own 'duty' – to lose weight. His sister, a nurse, has stood up for him, refusing to keep telling him that he's liable to have a heart attack at any moment. Sadly, the family regard her as a traitor.

Unlike fat women (who enjoy some hormonal protection against heart disease until they reach the menopause) fat men have to face up to the fact that their weight does pose an increased risk of heart attack. Research has suggested that men whose extra weight is distributed around the stomach area (rather than all over) are especially at risk.

On the other hand, weight is not the only risk factor in heart disease. Stress can play a significant role too. It is one thing to make a fat man aware of the risks he faces, and quite another to bully him and scare him out of his wits, as Diana points out.

Body size isn't a clearcut moral issue. Even if it was in some way this man's 'fault', that would not justify the way in which his family are trying to punish him. As it happens, the problem is not even of his making. He is labelled morally lacking, greedy and self-indulgent because of a series of disastrous childhood diets. And while one half of the world expects him to feel guilty and miserable about his size, you can be sure that the other half expects him to conform to the old 'fat and jolly' stereotype.

Not all fat men worry about their weight. Comedian Les Dawson takes a relaxed approach these days, despite a health scare in 1988:

> First of all doctors look at your weight. They looked at my stomach and said I'd have to diet. Lose weight, don't drink and don't smoke. All you can do is what you think is right – so I didn't do anything. Though I did give up smoking.

He takes a cynical view of diets:

> Appearances matter to everybody, so what you do is buy a suit that's slightly too small, and people say 'You look a mess'. Then you buy another suit that fits, but is a bit too big. Now the doctor says 'You've listened. You've been on the F-Plan. . . . You are getting thin, and to be thin today means being healthy.' The third suit has to be enormous, preferably with an enormous hat. Then the doctor says 'You've gone too far! Get some steak and chips down you right now' (talking on *Wogan*, BBC1, 1989).

John is a food and drink columnist. He is also fat, and readily admits that the two are linked: 'I eat and drink far more than is good for me.' Nowadays, John is happy with his size and describes himself as a 'professional fat man'. But it wasn't always so:

> About 15 years ago I did diet and got down to a fighting weight, but I found I was full of aches and pains, and whenever there was a 'flu bug in town I'd be the first to get it. . . . So what I decided to do was develop a three-dimensional 'fat personality', on the grounds

that I could conform to a group. I asked myself 'What are fat men like? – they're like Orson Welles and Peter Ustinov.' So I decided *I* was going to be like Orson Welles and Peter Ustinov – people who've made a success at 'fatness'; people who are fat and don't give a damn.

Some would call this an irresponsible attitude to take: doesn't John worry about the health risks of his 'eat, drink and be merry' lifestyle? He replies defiantly:

This fat business has less to do with health and heart attacks than with image. . . . Fat in itself is just another manifestation of all the things we're supposed to be – 'norms'. Thin is one of them. One of my friends, who shares my tastes in food and opera, says that I have to be fat, because otherwise I just wouldn't look right.

According to John, a fat man's problems have as much to do with psychological pressures as with practical considerations:

The only miserable fat people are people who'd prefer to be thin. People who want to be thin and aren't are just trying desperately to conform. But I've always had a sneaking suspicion that if *everyone* does something it's probably wrong.
  If a man wants to be thin, it's no problem. It can be done. In fact, I've done it. But if you look at Middle Eastern countries, for example, fat has a great deal to do with being desired. Society has an image. Everything you do is circumscribed by what you think you *ought* to do. Every time you see an advertisement, the image is always wrapped around a thin person. Because I'm reasonably tall I feel I can afford not to worry too much about it. But if I were short I might feel differently . . . I think short, fat men have the worst time of all.

Trouble really starts, according to John, when what we are doesn't match up with what we think we ought to be – and becomes an obsession:

Your self-image is a combination of what you think you are and what you'd like to be. Some people are what they think they ought to be, which is fun. Some aren't, but don't give a damn – and that's fun too. If I take someone who's happy with their size out to lunch, at least they can enjoy it: they're not going to order lettuce and

71

mineral water. . . . At the end of the day we have to examine our motives. It's like the child who wants a bigger paintbox because his friend's got a bigger paintbox. We have to ask ourselves: are we individuals, or are we conformists?

John admits that not everyone would agree with his defiant outlook on life – though it has clearly worked wonders for *his* own self-confidence. But is John one of a tiny minority? Are there other men who share his attitude to size?

One big man definitely to be reckoned with is TVam's astrologer, Russell Grant, who describes himself as 'Happy with my size 75% of the time'. Russell has not always been large. It was not until he gave up smoking and drinking that he began to put on weight. He now weighs around 15 stone.

He recognises that there are drawbacks in being a large man, though he feels that 'being big is the same for both men and women. Most people, seeing my size, think I must be happy all the time. It's as though I'm not allowed to be down. My size does affect my life in some ways – the main cons being the difficulty of finding clothes that fit, and the effects on my health. My size has also stopped me from doing some of the sports that have interested me, though of course that may be just a convenient excuse!'

It may seem ironic – in a world where television and skinniness are so closely linked in people's minds – but on the whole, Russell feels that his size has worked in his favour: 'A plus has been the positive effect it has had on my public image,' he explains. There seems little doubt that his size has been one factor in getting him noticed and helping to create his considerable public following.

Russell has no time for those who try to exert pressure on large people to change the way they look: 'My advice to people unhappy about their size would be to be yourself,' he says. 'Don't listen to what others would have you do and be. People seldom advise me to diet. If they do, I feel they should mind their own business.'

An article in *The Observer* ('It's the 16st laugh-in', 30 April 1978) took the publication of *Fat is a Feminist Issue* as an ideal opportunity to examine men's attitudes to their weight. 'Plump men,' asserted Vicki Mackenzie, 'seem to have a blind spot when it comes to self appraisal. Fat and happy is a phrase they embrace without even a sideways look at their girth in the mirror.' She noted that only 5 per cent of Weight Watchers members were men (although men tend to lose weight more successfully than women), and suggested 'Men don't *diet*; they go into training.'

The men she interviewed – a butcher, an accountant and actor Christopher Biggins – all agreed with her theories. In fact, they were positively defiant. The actor was photographed wearing a scarf with the legend 'Biggins is Beautiful'. Life, said the men, just wasn't worth living without a good meal and a few drinks. Anyhow, they had never had any problems attracting sexual partners, so why worry? The butcher went one step further: 'They say beer kills your sex life but when you've had a few you couldn't care less.'

A survey conducted on a sample of three is hardly scientific, but there's no doubt about it: the modern world is a confusing place for fat men.

Images of fat men: Mr Atlas meets the Bunter syndrome

Since Vicki Mackenzie wrote her article, the climate has changed. Advertisements for slimming meals show lean young men exchanging banter with lean young women as they sit down to a plate of low-fat white meat and lightly cooked vegetables. Advertisements for sunflower margarine play on male worries about cholesterol. It's difficult to be big and jolly when everyone is telling you how unhealthy you look.

The culpability trap, which has so long affected women, is now gaping wider and wider for fat men too. The new message is clear: fat is bad, greedy, lazy, apathetic, stupid, ugly, feeble and sexually questionable. The old tradition – that big is strong, healthy, jolly, desirable and masculine – refuses to die but is having a hard time to hold its own. Mr Atlas has his back up against the wall.

Light relief?

'I could never be a straight man – I'm the wrong shape' (Eddie Large)

One of the oldest humorous images we know is that of the fat, jolly man. Falstaff – everyone's idea of a fat man – said: 'I am not only witty in myself, but the cause that wit is in other men.' We may laugh at a man because his physical shape seems ridiculous to us, the exaggerated embodiment of a host of secret vices, but the fat man is also often gifted with a powerful wit.

Perhaps this is because fat boys learn at school that one good way to deflect bullying and criticism is to become a clown: to laugh at themselves and to make jokes. The fat man may appear jolly, but the role he plays is imposed on him by his appearance. Take Oliver Hardy, for example – he was deeply sensitive about his weight, and never quite got over the shock of being ridiculed in an Army recruiting office in 1917.

G. K. Chesterton is another case in point. He was extremely fat (over 135 kg, 300 lbs) but also extremely active, giving the lie to the idea that all fat men are lazy and stupid; he wrote over 100 books. Nevertheless, despite his great sense of humour, Chesterton was unhappy about his size. In typical, self-deprecating mood he once commented: 'Why, only yesterday on the Underground I had the pleasure of offering my seat to three ladies.' Modern alternative comedian Alexei Sayle introduces his show with a cruel, self-mocking parody of the Mickey Mouse theme song: 'Who's an ugly bastard, and as fat as he can be? – A–L–E–X–E–I S–A–Y–L–E.'

Billy Bunter is the traditional fat scapegoat, the embodiment of every negative quality ever associated with being fat. Bunter is greedy, unintelligent, dishonest, cowardly, feeble, clumsy – and exceedingly fat. He is shortsighted, his clothes are too tight and he speaks in a squeaky voice. We laugh at him because he is everything we believe we are not. In laughing, we express our alienation. We drive him out, like a devil.

Billy Bunter did not start out life as the avaricious, slothful, contemptible character we know so well. In the beginning, he was simply fat and generally amiable. But it wasn't long before he became the villain of the piece – a lower middle-class misfit in a world of princes and aristocrats, a fat failure in an atmosphere of svelte success. There are other 'baddies' at Greyfriars – boys who steal, tell tales, bet on the horses, and dissipate their youth in a cloud of clandestine cigarette smoke. But none has the tragi-comic stature of Billy Bunter – in every sense a 'rounded' character.

It can be no coincidence that Billy Bunter is one of the few instantly recognizable characters in C. H. Chapman's illustrations. With the exception of the token coloured boy – Indian aristocrat Hurree Jamset Ram Singh – the other members of the Remove are near-identical in appearance – as anodyne as characters in a 1950s toothpaste advertisement.

Bunter is in every respect different from his peers. His rotundity, his lower middle-class background, his owlish spectacles, his tight check trousers all mark him out as an outcast. Since he is almost always pictured on the end of someone's boot, flat on his back in the quadrangle or sneaking out of Wharton's study with a fruitcake tucked under his arm, there can be no doubt that Bunter is intended to evoke laughter, derision and perhaps a little pity. His fatness is like a signpost, saying 'Laugh at me – I'm different.'

The *Viz* character Tubby Johnson is another case in point. Tubby has one vice – he is a glutton, his favourite food is lard – so of course he is also extremely fat. Like Bunter he is shown as the face of hopeless, culpable weakness.

But fat men can be funny without being ridiculous. In fact, they need not be funny at all – images can be changed. Actor/writer Robbie Coltrane is never mocked for his size. He can be funny, menacing, magnificent – and sexy. He has tremendous acting ability and writes wonderful material which takes no account of anyone else's preconceptions. His success must also be due to his great self-assurance. He is never in any doubt as to his worth. He challenges the world to put him down – but who would dare to try?

Media men

The ranks of the famous include many successful fat men. Fine actors like Sidney Greenstreet, Orson Welles, John Candy, Raymond Burr and William Conrad – all of them respected for their acting ability and owing much of their success to their size.

Yet simply being famous is not a guarantee of happiness with one's size. This is especially true of men who have not always been fat. Take Marlon Brando. His considerable weight gain over the last few years has provoked a mixture of embarrassment and amusement in the world's press, somehow devaluing his standing as an actor.

On 17 September 1989, *SunDay* magazine ran a feature entitled 'From Raunchy to Paunchy', in which actors Corbin Bernsen, Jack Nicholson, Roger Moore and Michael Douglas were described as the 'Flab Four'. Full of puns and unflattering photographs, the article contains captions such as 'the Joker's become the Porker! He got a nice fat fee for Batman – but now Jack can be called Fatman.' The entire piece is about weight. Just because four middle-aged actors have put on a little weight, they are paraded before us as failures. The obsession with having a perfect shape is beginning to affect men as well as women.

The same thing happened to Henry (The Fonz) Winkler, former star of 'Happy Days'. Rather than highlight Winkler's success as a film producer and director, the magazine arrived at the banner headline 'I'm 44, fat and living in fear' (*SunDay*, 29 October 1989). 'Fat' turns out to consist of a smallish paunch and a double chin which is as much due to age as to size. His 'fear' is a vague anxiety about the problems of the world – and the 'love handles' around his waistline. Interestingly, the piece could be reworked as a success story, but 'fat sensationalism' triumphs.

Like fat women, all fat men are potential media targets. Some even court publicity. When 'massive motorist' Jack Galinsky bought the personalized number plate 'FAT BOY', he made sure *The Sun* was there to record the occasion and photograph his 'bulky bodywork' (23 October 1989). And *The Sport* – always first on the scene with a story about body size – wrote gleefully about the 'Globfather' – their name for a 360 kg (57 stone) American drug dealer who had to be moved to jail by forklift truck (16 April 1989).

Fat is not always grotesque or undesirable, even in the press. In December 1989, *Elle* magazine published a feature on American singer/songwriter Barry White, entitled 'Luurve!'. Writer Sally Brampton was mesmerized by the 'cult King of Love':

> Barry White is a gentleman. He is also a big boy. A very big boy. Six feet six with a girth that no laydee could get her arms around and a voice as big and sweet and deep as an earthquake rolling through honey. Seismic. The Voice of Sex.

Granted, Barry White has his height on his side (if he was 1.5 m (5 feet) tall, would he still be a sex symbol?) and of course that distinctive gravelly voice. But a sex symbol? There is no denying the fact that Mr White is not just big: he is also fat. Perhaps his success lies in his uncompromising self-confidence. Like Robbie Coltrane, he will admit of no doubt about himself. His outrageous chauvinism is just another part of his immense and very macho personality. He may be big, but there's no way Barry White will ever be a victim.

Can fat be invisible?

Must a fat man always be remembered as a fat man, rather than as a clever man or a successful one? Or can the problems associated with being big be overcome?

Over the years, society has become more and more confused about its attitude towards big men. A health-conscious culture like ours places a huge amount of responsibility on the individual for the care and maintenance of his or her own body. As early as the 1880s, one male writer was hinting that obesity should be made a criminal offence because it was a form of suicide (see p. 42). So the fat man bears a terrible weight of guilt and anxiety on his shoulders.

On the other hand, amid talk about the Danes imposing a tax on fat workers and managers being sacked for not losing enough weight, we still have our larger-than-life heroes and success stories. There are fat tycoons, fat politicians, and fat celebrities; there are fat Mensa members and fat Mastermind contestants to prove us wrong if we suggest that fat means unintelligent; and there are plenty of fat general practitioners to raise our eyebrows at when they tell us to lose weight.

There will always be fat men, thin men and all sorts of sizes in between. The essence of life is variety. The best size to be is the one with which you are comfortable, healthy and happy. In the second half of this book, we shall look at a variety of possible ways to achieve a better self-image and quality of life.

One fat man who has made a great success of his life is MP Sir Cyril Smith. Adored by his constituents in Rochdale and respected by politicians of every party, Sir Cyril has achieved a personal reputation which any statesman – fat or thin – would envy.

Sir Cyril – who is 1.9 m (6′2½″), weighs 180 kg (29 stone) and has a 160 cm (64″) waist – admits that life for a fat man can be fraught with problems:

> I have to have all my clothes made – including my underwear – because I can't buy anything off the peg. In fact, I'm having a pair of shoes made for me at the moment, for the first time. Seating is also a problem: the stability causes me concern. You don't show it, but you're a bit worried in case it collapses.

Theatre seats with iron arms, Tube barriers, football turnstiles and public toilets are all facilities that Sir Cyril would like to change.

> British Rail toilets on trains cause me a lot of problems. To try and get through that door, it's like trying to squeeze a sardine into a tin that's already full. Absolutely hopeless. Aeroplanes too. You tend to try and discipline yourself so that you don't need to use the services, because of the problems. I've been lucky in that I've never had to pay for two aircraft seats, though I suspect that's because of who I am. The air hostesses have always tried, without my saying a word, to make sure that the seat next to me was left vacant.

I think more provision should be made. The fact is that a tremendous emphasis has been put on disability in this country over the last ten or fifteen years. What most people fail to realize is that obesity is in itself a disability. They cater for the man with one leg, or the man with one eye, and quite rightly so, but they tend to overlook the necessity to cater in disabled terms for the obese.

Although he regards his size as a disability, Sir Cyril has never allowed it to stop him doing what he wanted to do. On the few occasions when he has had adverse reactions from the public, he has shrugged off the insult:

like water off a duck's back. I either laugh at it, ignore it or return the insult. The best way to deal with jokes is to laugh with them – don't let them offend you. Tell them to get stuffed occasionally – but in a humorous way. Of course, the cruellest people are children, but it's innocent cruelty with them.

He believes that big men *can* be fit and healthy 'though you wouldn't try to run a marathon'. He says that since he turned 60 the strain is beginning to tell on his knee joints, but he claims to have given up dieting because 'I lose 20, 25 or even 30 kg (3, 4 or 5 stone) and then I get fed up. I suppose I might have another go sometime, but I like eating.'

Sir Cyril's view of life is an overwhelmingly positive one. As far as his career is concerned, he is convinced that his size has helped rather than hindered him:

As a matter of fact, I think I'm taken more seriously as a politician than I would be if I were thin, because I'm noticed: I'm different from anybody else. The media certainly notice you when you're big, so you get a lot of attention that you would not otherwise get. On occasions, I play up to it. You're expected to be jolly, to take a joke – which I can – but the fact that you're easily recognized is a great help, politically. . . . There is nothing to be depressed about, as far as size is concerned. I have no doubt at all that big people can be both healthy and attractive. Brains have no direct relevance to size. Most good occupations can be filled by large people as well as not-so-large people. I don't see any reason to feel in any way embarrassed about being large. Beauty is only skin deep and we all have our good features – everybody's beautiful in their own way. Just get on with life, and take it all in your stride.

Summing up

Leaning to accept yourself as you are can only be achieved in easy stages. Here are a few areas on which you could try working:

- recognizing that you are more than just your body
- recognizing that body size does not affect your worth as a warm, intelligent, successful and sexual man
- challenging stereotypes: and accepting that you can choose *not* to play the clown or the scapegoat
- refusing to allow your size to rule your life
- talking to other men to promote greater understanding. To quote John, a 'medium large' man, 'Men don't easily have the same sense of sister/brotherhood as women do, so what we need are more men's groups – not fat men's groups, just men's groups.'

A parting shot

The next time you feel down about your weight, you might like to remember this apocryphal story:

> Two men were travelling on a bus – one thin, one fat. The thin man turned to the fat man and said, haughtily, 'I really think the bus company ought to charge according to weight.'
>
> 'Indeed?' replied the fat man. 'Well they wouldn't bother to pick you up.'

Further reading

Magna (magazine for big and tall men)
Box 286
Cabin John
MD 20818
USA

'Architecture of the Body', in *A History of Women's Bodies*, Edward Shorter (London: Pelican, 1984)
Fat and Thin, Anne Scott Beller (1980)

5

Big, Beautiful and Fit?
The Great Health Debate

Is it possible to be big and healthy, fat and fit? That is the question to which we would all love to know the answer. But it isn't just a matter of a simple yes or no.

Most doctors believe that big is by definition unhealthy. This goes hand in hand with the idea of culpability which we discussed in an earlier chapter. Being big isn't just a fact of life – it's something about which we are supposed to feel guilty and try to change.

But it's not that easy. There is no doubt that certain disorders (such as high blood pressure) can be exacerbated by being very large, but current research seems unwilling to oblige our prejudices by turning up a simple correlation between obesity and mortality or general illhealth. The issues are complex, confusing and frequently acquire inappropriate moral overtones.

What is fat?

Not every big person is fat, and not every fat person is particularly big. If that sounds nonsensical, think of all those Olympic shot-putters and hammer-throwers. They may be overweight by insurance standards, but they're not overfat. Their bulk is largely made up of muscle growth and bone. It is possible to be thinner and yet 'fatter' – that is, for a higher proportion of your body to be made up of fat – and therefore potentially less fit.

Statistics suggest that the fattest group of people in Britain today are middle-aged working-class women, aged 40 to 59, 73 per cent of whom are said to be overweight. This figure decreases to 49 per cent among middle-aged upper class women, and among young upper-class women the figure is only 27 per cent. Men tend to be leaner overall, though around 53 per cent of middle-aged middle-class men are overweight: a result of expense account lunches, perhaps? (Nikki Knewstub, *Guardian*, 9 April 1980).

We all have some body fat, of course – but what is it, and why do some of us have much more than others?

Fat is nature's store-cupboard – an emergency reserve for hard times. It insulates our bodies and provides a pool of ready energy when food is scarce. Women are intended by nature to carry greater fat stores than men, to enable them to survive through pregnancy and nursing if times are difficult.

Fat is kept in liquid form inside special fat cells, around half of which are just under the skin (subcutaneous fat). When we take in less food than we need, fat is burned to produce energy, and the cells shrink. If we eat more than we need, the surplus is stored and the cells inflate.

Your fat reserves are not inert. Even if your intake of food exactly matches your energy output, fat is continually being synthesized (made) and degraded (broken down). The continual breakdown of fat produces byproducts (free fatty acids) which enter the bloodstream and the liver.

Everyone needs fat: it's just a question of how much. Since the beginning of this century, life assurance tables have provided a norm against which we can measure the 'acceptability' of our bodies. By insurance standards, around a third of all Britons are at least 10 per cent overweight and 3 per cent are judged 'medically obese' (this would mean that someone who ought to weigh 60 kg (10 stone) actually weighed 80 kg, 13 stone).

Yet actuarial tables are a harsh judge of body size, and many researchers now suspect that they are pitched too low. While – on average – we have all got taller and fatter in recent years, insurance tables have actually been revised downwards. More and more of us are finding ourselves classified as 'moderately obese' – a mysterious category which did not even exist until a few years ago. To dare to step beyond the bounds of 'acceptable' size is, we are told, courting early death. But recent research is raising some interesting questions and challenges that may yet persuade insurance companies to take a more flexible view.

Why isn't everyone fat?

Traditionally, experts have tended to explain away the greater incidence of working-class obesity as the result of poor diet and education. However, one recent controversial theory has suggested that class – and body size – tend to be inherited. According to this American theory, working-class women tend to be fatter because their ancestors suffered repeated starvation and only those who had been the fattest were able to survive. Therefore their descendants have inherited their greater than average tendency to put on weight.

Whether or not we subscribe to this view, it has to be said that some of us do have a greater potential to be larger than others. In the late 1940s, a Frenchman called Vague suggested that human beings can be divided into three body types:

- ectomorphs
- mesomorphs
- endomorphs

Ectomorphs have long limbs and long, narrow hands and feet. These are the people who drive everyone else mad because they can apparently eat as much as they like and never put on weight. Most fat people are endomorphs: that is, they have short, squat figures, a large body and short arms and legs. According to Vague's theory, this is the body type most prone to obesity. Somewhere in the middle are the 'mesomorphs'.

Dr R. Barron once remarked that there are no fewer than 25 different ways of provoking weight gain in laboratory animals – so why should the human body be any different? Certainly experts have come up with a wide variety of possible causes to date.

Heredity

If you have large parents, your chances of being large are greatly increased. A child with two thin parents has only a 1 in 10 chance of being fat. With one large parent, the chance increases to almost 50–50. With two large parents, the child has only a 1 in 5 chance of *not* being fat (quoted in Weigall, 'The Fat of the Land', *The Listener*, 28 February 1974). Twins tend to resemble each other and adopted children take after their natural parents in size and shape – not their adoptive parents. So we have to question the belief that obesity results solely from bad eating habits – though it would be foolish to deny that there are fat people who do have a disturbed relationship with food.

Slow metabolic rate

Many people believe that obesity is simply the result of overeating. This may be so in many cases – but what exactly *is* overeating? One person's nutritional needs can be very different from another's. Some people can exist on just a few hundred calories a day (the equivalent of, say, one sandwich) without losing weight. For them, enjoying a 'normal' diet means putting on weight. If they want to remain thin, they have to contend with a lifetime of hunger and deprivation.

Hormones

Some people become fat because of an endocrine (hormone) imbalance.

'Environmental' factors

Sometimes obesity can be caused by, for example, immobilization during illness or accident.

Eating disorders

There is a tendency to assume that all fat people – especially women – suffer from eating disorders. Perhaps some people believe that this is a charitable view – excusing what they perceive to be gluttony on the grounds that it is the result of some deep-seated emotional problem.

Not surprisingly, most fat people see red when they encounter this attitude. Not only is it patronizing: it is also inaccurate. Repeated research into obesity has failed to prove that fat people are excessive eaters. In fact, it has shown that the average fat person is 'euphagic' that is to say that he or she eats about the same as the average thin person. In some cases, the fat person even eats less than his or her thin friend. The truth is that there are both fat and thin people who overeat or who eat a poorly balanced diet; but the majority of fat people are not gluttons.

The eating disorders that most people think of are anorexia nervosa (compulsive self-starvation) and bulimia nervosa (in which the sufferer binges, then vomits or takes huge doses of laxatives in order to avoid digesting the food). Logic would suggest that most sufferers stay thin, since they either starve themselves or rid themselves of the food they eat before they have a chance to digest it.

Susan Howard, a psychologist, concluded that people with eating disorders may be thin or fat, but that in either case they are likely to be chronic dieters: 'Not one woman in my study had binged before she began to diet' (*Extra Special*, April/May 1988). So it would seem that in pressurizing people to become thin, we may also be promoting that unnatural fixation with food which comes from starvation or deprivation.

Trauma

In rare cases, a physical injury can lead to weight gain. One example of this would be damage to a part of the brain called the hypothalamus, which is involved with feelings of hunger and fullness. Damage can disrupt these signals, leading either to starvation or to voracious, uncontrolled eating.

In most people, body size will depend not just on what we eat, but on our genetic make-up. Many experts now believe that each individual body has its own 'setpoint': a natural weight that it will attempt to maintain. Some of us are 'meant' to weigh more than the insurance companies want us to weigh, and if we want to be thinner we will have to fight our bodies all the way. Others (the ectomorphs) may find themselves struggling not to be 'underweight'. Very few of us find it easy to be 'perfect'. The question is: should we continue to try?

Is fat harmful to health?

There is no doubt that some medical conditions are linked to obesity, though the link is not necessarily as simple as it seems. High blood pressure, adult onset diabetes and coronary heart disease are at the top of the scale of diseases about which large men and women worry. Over the years, doctors have also suggested links with arterial disease, stroke, arthritis, accidental and sudden death, surgical problems, kidney failure, infertility and mental problems such as shyness, hysteria and overassertiveness.

It's quite a burden of guilt to bear. But before you go on another crash diet, let's take a closer look at the facts.

A death sentence?

The popular belief is that fat people do not live as long as thin people – in fact Hippocrates was saying so as early as the fourth century BC. But modern research is questioning the old assumptions.

Paul Ernsberger has made an extended study of the evidence over a period of years, and is not convinced by the insurance charts or a recent National Institute of Health study which dubbed obesity a 'killer disease'. Ernsberger looked carefully at the following studies.

The Seven Country Study (1960–75)

Around 13 000 middle-aged men were weighed and observed for fifteen years. Surprisingly enough, the highest death rate turned out to be among those men who had started out as the leanest, while the lowest death risk was for the moderately fat. The very fat carried a greater risk than the merely plump, but – amazingly – it was still lower than the risk for the very thin. This study dismissed insurance tables as unreliable.

The Norway Study

Here 1.8 million people were followed for a period of ten years. Once again, the highest death risk turned out to be among those who were 'underweight'. The lowest rate proved to be for those who were around 30 per cent overweight by insurance standards. After this point, death rates increased gradually but were still *lower* than those for the underweight.

According to Dr Ernsberger, it may well be safest to be around 10–30 per cent heavier than the figures quoted by insurance companies. Yet even for those who are heavier still, it is not all doom and gloom. He gives the example of a very thin fashion model and a plump, 'queen-size' model. If the underweight woman loses ¼ kg (1 lb) in weight, she increases her risk of dying by around 1 per cent. Yet if her 'queen-size' colleague puts on ¼ kg (1 lb), her risk increases by only 0.1 per cent.

Another well-respected American expert – Dr Reubin Andres, of the National Institute of Aging – led a major review of the available evidence, which concluded that: 'the (16) major studies of obesity and mortality fail to show that overall obesity leads to greater risk'. (*Radiance*, Winter 1986).

Enough to make your blood boil?

Although some diseases are more common among fat people, Dr Ernsberger points out that there are no diseases which affect *only* fat people. In fact, some diseases are much more common in thin people. Next time you are feeling low, you can always console yourself with the fact that you are less likely than a thin person to suffer from:

- osteoporosis (the brittle bone disease that strikes many thin women in their later years); fat women produce more oestrogen, which protects both against this condition and against premature ageing. (On the negative side, an excess of oestrogen can in rare cases have a detrimental effect on fertility.)
- some forms of cancer (though on the negative side, fat women have an *increased* incidence of uterine cancer)
- some lung diseases (for example emphysema).

New research into hypertension (high blood pressure) has raised the question of whether it is a disease of failed dieters rather than a disease of fat people. Hardening of the arteries, leading to heart attack and stroke, can also be linked to repeated dieting (*Obesity and Health*, 1966, quoted in V. F. Mayer, 'The Fat Illusion', *Shadow on a Tightrope*, p. 9).

Experiments carried out on laboratory rats showed that, although these animals do not generally suffer from high blood pressure, they developed the condition after repeated cycles of starving and regaining weight. In the end, they appeared to have developed permanent hypertension and their heart function was also affected, possibly by the production of a stress hormone called noradrenaline.

The process is thought to be similar in humans. When you starve yourself, and begin to lose weight, your blood pressure falls. But if, as most dieters do, you put all or some of the weight you have lost back on again, your blood pressure may rise *beyond* its original level. So, according to Ernsberger, chronic failed dieting could be one cause of hypertension.

A study published in 1980 by a team led by R. T. Jung indicated that the fall in blood pressure from three weeks' stringent dieting was obliterated after only three days of moderately low-calorie eating ('The effect of refeeding after starvation on catecholamine and thyroid metabolism', *International Journal of Obesity*, 4:95, 1980).

Another recent development in health research is the question of fat distribution. In his article, 'Fat is a positional issue' (*The Guardian*, 24 July 1987) Michael Gibney (a nutrition expert from Trinity College Medical School, Dublin) suggests that it is your *shape* rather than your *size* that determines your chances of leading a healthy life.

This new theory challenges the methods used by doctors to determine whether or not a patient is overweight, and questions whether or not they can also be used to calculate the health risks that the patient faces.

Most doctors calculate obesity using the *body mass index* (BMI), which is worked out as follows:

$$\frac{\text{weight in kilograms}}{(\text{height in metres})^2}$$

However, according to Michael Gibney, studies in Gothenburg and Paris have challenged the BMI as an indicator of health risk. Researchers now believe that the waist : hip circumference (WHC) ratio is a much better predictor of coronary heart disease and diabetes risk. The WHC ratio enables doctors to determine if a patient's obesity follows an 'android' or 'gynoid' pattern. Android obesity is a typical 'male' shape, with large belly, small bottom and thighs. Gynoid obesity is typical of many women, with slender waist, neat abdomen, large bottom and heavy thighs. Apparently it is the android form that carries the greater risk, and that is why the WHC ratio is important. The larger the waist is in relation to the hips, the more 'android' the obesity –and the greater the health risk.

This would explain why fat is generally agreed to be a greater health risk for men than it is for women, though it also suggests that women whose obesity takes the 'android' form may be at equal risk. Fat from all areas of the body is continually broken down, producing degradation products called free fatty acids. The way in which these are dealt with by the body depends on the area from which they come, and experts believe that fatty acids from abdominal fat are more harmful to the body than those coming from the bottom or thighs.

In android (abdominal) obesity, free fatty acids flow directly to the liver via the hepatic portal vein, and the level of these acids in the liver tends to be high. This can impair the liver's ability to inactivate insulin, leading to high levels of blood insulin – a typical feature of adult-onset diabetes, which is often associated with obesity, and itself increases the risk of coronary heart disease. High blood insulin may also lead to raised blood pressure. There is some evidence that high levels of blood fats (which are packaged in the liver) may be linked to the high inflow of fatty acids into the liver – and a high blood-fat count is another risk factor in coronary heart disease.

In short, it now looks as if the risk of coronary heart disease is greatly increased in android obesity. This is largely due to the different physiological properties of fat stores in different parts of the body. In general, it is good news for women and bad news for men. As one expert concludes: 'If you're fat, be fat all over.'

One last consideration in the great health debate is the role of stress and anxiety. We all know that stress is a risk to our health, and that it can be a factor in the development of high blood pressure. Yet we tend to underestimate the extent to which large people may feel stressed by other people's negative opinions of them. The few surveys that have been carried out in societies where fat is acceptable have suggested that fat people may be a lot healthier when they do not feel persecuted.

Exercise

There is evidence to suggest that fat people are less physically active than their thin peers. This is probably why 'fat' has become synonymous with 'lazy' and 'apathetic'.

Many people believe that the lack of exercise makes people fat.

Others believe that people stay fat because they do not exercise. Studies of college students in America have shown that fat adolescent girls are indeed less active than their peers – but they have also shown, interestingly, that the fat girls eat *less* than their slim colleagues. It could be that they are inactive because they have little energy.

Perhaps the main reason for inactivity is embarrassment about body size. Some fat people believe that they cannot exercise, or that if they do, they will be mocked by slim people. Others give up trying to exercise because they cannot find suitable sportswear in their size.

Large people can – and should be allowed to – enjoy physical exercise which is geared to their size and personal capabilities, exercise which is gentle and sensible and fun. Exercise will not make you thinner, but it can tone you up and make your heart and lungs stronger. In the next chapter we shall talk about ways in which you can discover exercise yourself; it need not be just for thin people.

Doctors' attitudes

As we have seen in an earlier chapter, doctors' attitudes are a real problem for many fat people. A high proportion of doctors take a punitive approach to dealing with their larger patients, adopting the philosophy that it's 'all for their own good'.

The trouble is that most general practitioners are so busy that they don't have time to read the latest research into obesity and health. Medical schools do not train them to take a sympathetic approach, and since they are only human they may sometimes allow their personal and cultural prejudices to affect the way they treat their patients.

Not all doctors are like this. Jenny, for example, has positive experiences to relate:

> My endocrinologist has been absolutely wonderful, and treats me like an intelligent woman. He respects my brain. He has made me feel that he cares about what's going wrong with my body, and has seen the effect rather than the cause to be the problem. He understands that I fight my body all the time.

Lee also has praise for her general practitioner:

> She's Asian, very good, never critical: she doesn't attribute every bout of bronchitis or whatever to my size. Another general practitioner (also Asian) once advised me not to worry about

losing weight, as he believed dieting all the time to be just as unhealthy as staying fat, if not more so.

At the other end of the scale is the 'lose 25 kg (4 stone) and call me in the morning' syndrome so familiar to many large patients. Helen Teague of Big Clothes recalls:

> We've got one customer who had a terrible back problem, and was off work for months. The doctor refused to treat her until she'd lost at least 44 kg (7 stone). She actually did lose the weight – but she's still got exactly the same back problem. It's no better. But at least the doctor will see her now.

Another woman recalls a bad experience in a maternity hospital: 'It was just the day after I'd had my baby. The sister walked past and thumped me in the stomach, and said "hold that in".'

This state of affairs is very worrying. If general practitioners refuse to treat their large patients as human beings, pretty soon none of them will be willing to put themselves through the agony any more. Who will go to see a doctor, knowing that the payoff is likely to be a humiliating lecture on slimming, second-class treatment and a heavy helping of sarcasm? We all deserve equal treatment, but it looks as if many of us are not getting it. A lot of the women I talked to have already forsaken mainstream medicine in favour of alternative therapists.

This is all very well, but when serious illnesses threaten we all need to feel we can call on the NHS. Elizabeth Osborne is well aware of the dangers:

> I don't usually go to see my general practitioner but on one occasion I had to, because I had skin cancer. I said, 'I am not going to be weighed. I am not coming to you about my weight, but about a mole on my face.' I really have to steel myself and make myself go, especially for cervical smears. You just know what they're thinking as you're lying there. And surgical gowns are a total embarrassment.

If patients become unwilling to consult a doctor about matters as serious as cancer, the implications are obvious. Many large patients are going to allow serious illnesses to go undetected. From a purely economic perspective this is nonsense, since an illness which could have been detected early on and cured cheaply and simply may well develop into an acute condition requiring expensive and lengthy in-patient care. Above all, it is wrong from a humanitarian point of view.

So what can you do to improve matters? Elizabeth suggests interviewing your prospective general practitioner before you sign on:

> I said, 'We will never discuss my weight unless we agree to. I will not be weighed unless we both agree that it is necessary. I don't want to be what you consider to be my ideal weight, but what I consider to be my ideal weight, which is heavier.' He was fine after that. You have to say, 'Do you realize how you are making me feel?' and 'Have you read the research?' I think the medical profession should be taught not to tell people they are fat and lazy.

If stress is bad for the health, then doctors should realize that unsympathetic treatment could in itself pose a health risk for their large patients. And the pressure that they exert on those patients are sometimes unjustifiably strong. One doctor who has recognized this is Dr Lorraine Bonner, a Californian general practitioner:

> She has found that studies do not separate the effects of weight from social oppression, or repeated cycles of weight loss and gain. Thus . . . it is difficult to know whether health problems are the result of being overstressed or overweight. . . . It is possible to be thin and have an eating disorder, or to be large and eat well (*Radiance*, Winter 1986).

Weighing up the risks

If you are moderately large, it's quite possible that you may also be fit and healthy. A great deal depends upon a number of interconnected factors:

- your family history
- smoking
- drinking
- the quality of your diet
- whether or not you exercise
- the level of stress in your lifestyle
- your shape (android or gynoid)
- your size (if you are *very* large this may carry an extra risk)

In deciding what to do with your life and with your body, you need to evaluate all these factors and determine what – if any – action you need to take in order to become healthier. If you are only moderately large, and your body size is your only risk factor, there is probably not too much to worry about. According to Professor Trevor Silverstone (an expert in human psychopharmacology), 'There is a high risk for the very, very obese, but it is not especially important for the moderately obese. . . . If obesity is a problem at all, it is in people's attitudes towards it' (Polly Toynbee, 'Fat and Happy?', *The Guardian*, 1 April 1985).

What price slenderness?

Dieting is a national sport of truly Olympic proportions. If we need any confirmation of the way in which it has captured our imaginations, we need only look at the way in which the diet products industry in the United Kingdom has grown over the last twenty years:

- 1969: worth £34 million
- 1979: worth £160 million
- 1989: worth £1 billion

It is estimated that around three-quarters of all seventeen-year-old girls in Britain are on diets; 250 000 girls and women are reckoned to have anorexia, with many more suffering from bulimia – and the latest news is that men are now suffering from anorexia, too. Faced with health and fashion propaganda, more and more of them are struggling to change their bodies.

Diet foods galore

A whole industry has sprung up to serve the dedicated dieter in his or her quest for the 'perfect' body.

Among the supermarket racks of 'Lean Cuisine' convenience meals (known apparently as 'Mean Cuisine' among rival manufacturers) are all the 'replacement' foods that have become a part of the dieter's existence. At the moment, sweeteners are the favourite artificial, low-calorie product. Next off the production line looks like being a fat replacement: the dieter's dream. At last! A calorie-free oil in which to fry chips! Doughnuts with artificial fat and sugar-free sweetener! But is it all as innocent as it seems?

Radio 4's 'Food Programme' (February 1990) announced that a major American manufacturer has now produced a calorie-free fat replacement (actually a sucrose polyester which behaves just like fat) called Alestra. It hasn't yet been approved for sale by the American Food and Drug Administration (there's some evidence that it causes pituitary tumours in rats), but the firm remain hopeful and the American public are clamouring to be allowed to buy the product. They aren't, apparently, worried about the quality of what they are putting into their bodies – but simply want the chance to eat low-calorie chips and cakes.

Also geared to the US market is the curiously named 'fluffy cellulose' – a bland fibre-based product apparently more suited to the American taste than the 'harsher' natural product, bran. As fluffy cellulose also serves to bulk out flour in bakery products, it can be used to reduce the calorific value of 'forbidden' foods like chocolate cake and sticky buns.

It sounds a good idea, but is it? Nutritionist Melanie Miller of the Consumers' Association, talking on the 'Food Programme', expressed considerable disquiet about these new 'replacements'. After all, if they become a common feature of our daily diet, how will we know the value and nutritional qualities of what we are eating? They might make you thinner, but they could also make you unhealthy. As she commented: 'People could suffer major malnutrition if these items form a large part of their diet.'

As long as we allow ourselves to perpetuate this hysterical quest for thinness, we will also encourage manufacturers to produce nutritionally worthless, expensive and maybe even harmful products to satisfy our taste for 'forbidden' foods.

The dieter's dilemma

Over the years, the desperate dieter has been presented with a baffling variety of weight-loss options, some of them positively harmful, some merely unpleasant. All of the following have been used by doctors in the United Kingdom or America, although many have undergone inadequate clinical trials:

- thyroid hormone (supposedly speeds up metabolism)
- injections made from the urine of pregnant women
- digitalis (a dangerous drug which acts on the heart)
- fasting
- massive doses of vitamins
- enemas ('colonic lavage')
- brain surgery
- jaw-wiring

- stomach stapling (gastroplasty)
- balloons inserted into the stomach
- intestinal bypass surgery
- low-calorie liquid diets
- dangerous appetite-suppressant drugs, including amphetamines (speed) – *highly addictive*

Ironically, while doctors have been supervising these dubious methods of weight reduction, they have been busily condemning those outside the medical sphere who have put forward their own solutions. One of the most notorious of these was the appalling Beverly Hills Diet: a regime guaranteed to make you want never to see another pineapple. One sufferer – a fifteen-year-old boy – wrote the following account of Ms Mazel's diet;

> I tried (it) for three days, and I felt absolutely AWFUL. And I don't think it was just the 'poisons' being flushed from my body. . . . You can't expect people to eat pineapples the whole time. One pineapple a day may keep the doctor away, but it also keeps you on the loo for most of the time. Perhaps that is the whole idea. In which case I've got better things to do with my day (*You Fat Slob!*, Anthony Palmer, 1985).

Unbelievably, that *was* the whole idea. The Beverly Hills Diet promoted weight loss by causing chronic diarrhoea, which would do you no good at all. If taken to extremes – in common with any high dose of laxative or diuretic – it could lead to an 'electrolyte' imbalance (loss of ions of potassium, calcium and magnesium) which might in turn lead to heart or kidney damage.

Any extreme 'fad' diet is likely to do you more harm than good, and even the most moderate diet can be agony to stick to. When you burn your fat reserves, free fatty acids enter the bloodstream and the hypothalamus (part of your brain) tries to persuade you to eat by creating terrible food fantasies. This is why you can't concentrate on your work, and can't stop thinking about chocolate éclairs all day long. It is also why balloons inserted in the stomach don't tend to be very effective: the hypothalamus knows you haven't eaten anything and continues to give you the food fantasies regardless.

Even if you do stick to a diet, the chances are that you'll eventually put all the weight back on. Research has shown that anything up to 99 per cent of all diets fail in the long term. Even the most optimistic estimates of success rates do not make very inspiring reading – and they are purely *short-term* successes:

- Weight Watchers: 30 per cent success
- general practitioners: claim a 12 per cent success rate
- dieting on own, without support: 1–12 per cent success rate
  (figures quoted from 'The Food Programme', Radio 4, February
  1990)

So why do we tend to put the weight back on so quickly? Researchers now believe that 99 per cent of diets are doomed to failure because our bodies are geared to maintain a certain weight. It's not so much a question of our weight being determined by what we eat, as eating instinctively for the weight which we are 'programmed' to maintain: the *setpoint*.

It is very difficult to alter your natural setpoint, either up or down. Regular vigorous exercise can lower it, but only a little. The minimal reduction produced by smoking simply isn't worth the risks of cancer, heart disease and respiratory complaints. Repeated crash-dieting tends to push the setpoint up, so that as soon as you stop dieting, you put all the weight back on – plus a bit extra. According to Susan Woolley, of the University of Cincinnati, a loss of 2.2 kg (5 lbs) virtually assured a regain of 2.7 kg (6 lbs). So if you are continually on and off diets you may end up weighing more than you would have done if you had never dieted at all.

The reason for this depressing fact of life seems to be that whenever you go on a crash diet, your body thinks that it is being deprived of food because there is a famine. So your metabolism slows down to make the best possible use of your energy reserves. When you start eating again, your body safeguards itself against the next 'famine' by putting on a bit of extra fat 'to be on the safe side'.

The only way to get round the problem is to get back in tune with your body, listen to its needs and so rediscover your natural setpoint. It may be higher than you would prefer, but at least you can maintain it and lose your terror of food. If your weight has risen and seems out of control, it can be reduced or at least stabilized through sensible, healthy eating. The most difficult part is having the courage to stop dieting and eat normal, regular, balanced meals again. Many fat women who do so are terrified that their weight will soar, but most find that they lose weight or at least put no more on. It's all about paying attention to hunger signals rather than calorie counts.

There are other side-effects of dieting of which every large person should be aware:

- rapid weight-loss may cause wrinkles and stretch marks

- you may lose muscle tissue as well as fat – and dead muscle cells cannot be renewed (don't forget the heart is made up of muscle tissue)
- most sufferers from eating disorders developed them after dieting.

Inadequate nutrition is an ever-present danger in very low-calorie diets, even ones like the Cambridge Diet which have been developed by scientists and are supposed to include all the essential vitamins and minerals.

One problem is that the diets are so low in calories that your body goes into 'starvation mode', and compensates for the lack of food by breaking down body tissues to produce energy. Unfortunately it isn't just fat that is broken down: you also lose protein from your bones, joints and muscles, and this has been known to have a weakening effect when diets are continued for more than a few weeks. In rare cases, the body's chemistry can be seriously disrupted.

There are also risks to consider even after you have finished the diet. Whenever you begin eating again after a fast or a low-calorie liquid diet, dangerous stresses are placed on your body, especially the cardiovascular system. In up to 95 per cent of all cases, there is a rapid regain of weight and this is *extremely hazardous* – leading in a few cases to heart problems and even sudden death.

Of course, we could maintain our new thinness by dieting for the rest of our lives, but to do so is to choose lifelong deprivation. Some people – mainly women – do choose this path because they prefer it to the jeers and catcalls they got when they were fat.

Others – for example, the members of the London Fat Women's Group – prefer to stop dieting, listen to their bodies' hunger and try to live with the 'setpoint' that nature has given them. That setpoint may be higher than society would like it to be, but at least their weight stabilizes and they are able to stop thinking about food all the time. And it doesn't mean abandoning yourself to massive weight gain. A couple of the women I spoke to who had given up dieting said that they had actually *lost* weight as a result – effortlessly.

The danger of eating disorders

One major problem with dieting is that it is a form of starvation and self-deprivation. Most of us like food, and when we are deprived of it we can think of little else.

The psychological mechanisms behind bulimia and anorexia are complex, but most people develop them after dieting. Surely it is better to be a large, healthy person with a natural relationship to food, rather than a thin, tormented person who binges and vomits?

Sufferers from anorexia and bulimia lose contact with their bodies' needs and may force themselves to vomit several times a day. Their throats swell from the constant scratching with fingernails, their teeth blacken and rot from stomach acid and their periods cease. They are no longer women but undernourished waifs with staring eyes.

The unkindest cut

Despite most people's horror of surgery, weight-reduction operations have grown in popularity over the last few years, especially in America. To some, they seem like the only hope after years of unsuccessful dieting. But do they work, and what is the price we pay?

You have to be pretty desperate to go through the agony of having your jaws wired together. In order to carry out this barbaric process, the dental surgeon must first grind down your teeth and then cover them with a special type of cement. Many patients find the whole process painful and degrading. When you walk down the street, people stare at the wires on your teeth. You can't talk properly or eat solid food, and you have to carry a pair of wirecutters around with you everywhere in case you choke on your own vomit.

Most people would baulk at the prospect. But not Janice. At 110 kg (18 stone) she felt she could take no more. She had her jaws wired and lost 5 stone in six months. As soon as the wires were taken off, she put it all back on again.

Then Janice heard about gastroplasty – the stomach stapling operation which leaves just a tiny part of your stomach so that you can eat minuscule meals. She had the operation on 26 October 1988, at Manchester Royal Infirmary: 'At times the pain was so great, I wondered whether I'd made a hideous mistake,' she admits. In seven months she lost 30 kg (5 stone) and she is still losing weight. But, sadly, all her enjoyment of food has disappeared. She can eat no more than a couple of spoonfuls without retching, and most days her sole food is a small bowl of soup. Is that living?

Other women have undergone intestinal bypass surgery, in which only a few metres or even centimetres of intestines are left to process food – hence most of it passes through the body, undigested. This can lead to a startling weight loss, but also causes explosive, painful diarrhoea and carries considerable danger of nutritional deficiency. Perhaps worst of all, this is a major surgical operation, carried out on a sound (if fat) body. It involves both pain and risk – and some people have died on the operating table, others later on because they didn't stop losing weight and simply couldn't face having the operation reversed.

Janice believes that it is only because of this operation that she is able to do all the things she has always wanted to do – ice skating, keep fit, dancing, going out – but really there is no reason why she could not have done these things before. Do we really have to undergo dangerous operations in order to make ourselves 'worthy' of living a full life? Must we risk our health in pursuit of a body that perhaps we were never meant to have?

The way ahead: putting quality back into your life

As we said in Chapter 4, obesity poses a greater risk for men than it does for women – especially for the very large man. On the plus side, men also seem to find it easier to lose weight and keep it off. Nevertheless, your size is not everything and it is worth assessing all your risk factors before embarking on a diet. If you do diet, make sure it's *slowly, steadily and sensibly* – and be sure that it's what you want, not something you're doing just to please someone else.

For women, the situation is rather different. A recent paper presented to the British Psychological Society suggested that most women are better off the way they are – and should only diet if medically obese. According to research psychologist Jane Ogden, seven out of ten women would be happier accepting themselves as they are, and casting off the belief that thinness is the key to success and the answer to every problem. After a supervised six-week diet, her 23 subjects all reported that their eating was out of control, that they thought of food all the time and wanted to binge.

If you are one of the seven out of ten, perhaps you should be thinking in terms of a new lifestyle, rather than a new diet. You need to learn how to:

- value yourself and recognize your needs
- reduce your stress and act with others to promote a more tolerant environment
- assert yourself, confront prejudice and promote a better understanding of your size
- resist medical discrimination and try to re-educate your doctor
- find social support through friends, relatives and groups (research suggests that this can itself give protection against some diseases like cancer)
- learn about nutrition and eat well
- evaluate your risk factors (smoking, weight, drink etc) and plan your lifestyle accordingly

- learn to relax
- take up gentle, fun, sustainable exercise.

Whether you lose weight or not is a side issue. The important thing is that you are escaping from the terrible food fixation that is so characteristic of diets, and setting your whole life on a new, healthier footing that you can sustain for the rest of your life.

If you need to lose weight for medical reasons, make sure that you do it gradually, healthily and under knowledgeable supervision. Don't just accept the usual diet sheet without complaint and resign yourself to failure yet again. Whether you decide to lose weight or to stay the way you are, remember: it's *your* body and it's *your* decision. Lose sight of that, and you really do lose control of your life.

Over the course of the next two chapters, we shall look at some of the ways in which you could work to improve the quality of your life – ways in which you can come to terms with your body and develop a better self-image. In Chapter 6, we talk about how your body looks and feels and how you can derive pleasure from looking after it. In Chapter 7, we move on to examine some of the social and mental skills which you can develop in order to gain a more positive and balanced attitude to life. The key to both chapters is acceptance: of the body you have now and not the body you may or may not have in six months' time.

Further reading

Shadow on a Tightrope, ed. Lisa Schoenfielder and Barb Wieser (originally published in America by Aunt Lute Press; available in the United Kingdom from Rotunda Press)
You Fat Slob, Anthony Palmer (London: Futura, 1985)

6

Caring for Your Body:
A Health Programme for Life

For many large people, health seems an irrelevant issue. 'How can I be fit and healthy?' they say. 'I'm so fat!' But as we saw in the previous chapter, the issues are not quite so clear-cut. Being very large *can* be a health risk if you also have other risk factors (such as smoking), but it is possible to be moderately big and healthy. You owe it to yourself to care for your body and help it to reach its full potential, *whatever your shape or size*.

In order to make the most of the body you have, you need to devise your own health programme, one which you know you can live by for the rest of your life. This isn't going to be another of those five-day grapefruit diets, high in deprivation and low in nutrition. By making subtle, comfortable changes in the way you live, you can show your body that you care. You need to:

- decide whether you intend to lose weight, or to live healthily at your present shape and size – the decision is yours, and no-one else's
- give your body the food it needs for health, energy and warmth
- give your body the exercise it needs for strength, stamina and suppleness.

Food for health

If you care about your body, you also care about what you put into it. People who accept and like themselves value good food because it makes them look and feel healthy – not because it helps them lose weight. If your body is a complex machine, think how important it is to give it the right fuel. You wouldn't try to run a Porsche on paraffin, so why upset your body's natural balance through faddy eating or junk food? Your body needs a subtle mix of nutrients, vitamins and minerals which it can only get from a balanced diet. Strange as it may seem, you don't have to be thin to suffer from malnutrition.

If, as many experts suspect, long-term crash dieting tends to make you fatter and disrupt your natural 'setpoint' mechanism (see page 94), it makes sense to opt for healthy food choices, rather than obsessive calorie-counting. Some nutrition experts believe that doing this can actually help you to regain your natural setpoint and perhaps lose a little weight as a result. This is borne out by several of the women I spoke to who had given up dieting and found – to their amazement –that they had got thinner rather than fatter. They had also escaped from the terrible food fantasies and obsessions that had haunted them throughout their dieting years.

Whatever the consequences may be in terms of your weight, you will have the satisfaction of knowing that you are doing what is right for your body. Sensible eating can be fun, and it certainly helps to minimize the health risks associated with being large. If, for example, you have a tendency to high blood pressure, it makes good sense to reduce your salt and fat intake. Even if you eat well already, the chances are that there's some room for improvement. Think about the following when you are doing the weekly shopping.

Salt

Experts recommend a daily sodium intake of around 4 g, but stress that this can be obtained from the salt already present in food: there is no need to add any extra. In fact, most of us consume too much – between 5 and 20 g daily.

Processed foods often contain much higher levels of salt than their fresh equivalents. For example, fresh pork contains around 63 mg of sodium per 100 g of meat, whereas for bacon the figure is 1480 mg! Kippers are a problem, too, with their 990 mg per 100 g (as opposed to 67 mg for fresh herring).

A surprise offender is the humble and ever-popular cornflake, which turns out to contain 1160 mg per 100 g. Not so surprising is that other breakfast-time favourite, Marmite, which tops our mini-poll with a spectacular sodium content of 4500 mg per 100 g.

These foods don't have to be cut out of your diet completely, but they shouldn't form a major part of it. If you stop adding extra salt to your meals, and take care to check the packaging on processed foods, avoiding the salt trap should be easy.

Fat

Most of us have got the message about fats and cholesterol, which – when eaten to excess – can increase the risks of arterial disease and certain cancers. It has been estimated that the average American consumes 40–45 per cent of his or her total calories in the form of fat. A healthy diet should contain perhaps 20 per cent fat, according to biomedical researcher Paul Ernsberger. Remember that many processed foods contain 'hidden' fats (so look at the labels) – a piece of salami could be 80 per cent fat! But don't forget the 'good guys' – the oils that are contained naturally in some fish such as herrings and mackerel, and which are thought to protect against heart disease. Doctors say we should eat these naturally oily fish at least once a week.

Sugar and white flour

These are highly processed foods that we don't really need and don't do us much good. Replace sugar with naturally sweet foods like fruit, and white flour with brown or stoneground.

Fibre

Nowadays, it's easy to increase your fibre intake because there are so many high-fibre products on the market, from breakfast cereals to brown bread. Don't forget that fresh vegetables are an important source of dietary fibre. Oats contain soluble fibre, which is thought to reduce levels of blood cholesterol in some people.

Starches

These are otherwise known as complex carbohydrates. For years, people have believed – *quite wrongly* – that foods such as potatoes, pasta, bread and rice are 'fattening'. Most doctors now recommend that these foods should be the mainstay of your diet. They are low in fat and a good source of sustained energy. Mind you, it's not a good idea to smother your pasta in cream or melted butter!

Treats

No matter how healthily we may try to eat, most of us have our dietary weaknesses – maybe chocolate, or fish and chips. If we existed entirely on these 'forbidden' foods, we would of course be pretty unhealthy. On the other hand, if we deny ourselves the occasional treat, we will never be able to stick to a lifelong healthy eating programme. Little by little, the spectre of the 'forbidden' jam rolypoly will loom up in our mind's eye until we can think of nothing else.

We have to learn that there are *no* forbidden foods, no foods that are entirely good or entirely bad – though some may be better for us than others. Self-denial is at the root of many eating disorders, so don't deny yourself. Treat yourself when you want to. If you listen to your body's hunger, and know that you can eat when you want whenever you want, the chances are that you won't want to eat chips all day long. Learn to respect your body, and you'll want to make sure that it gets the foods it needs for a healthy life.

Exploding the exercise myth

How did you feel about PE lessons when you were at school? Were you what Ann Harper calls 'the stereotypical fat non-athlete'? Unsympathetic teachers, unkind remarks by classmates and uncomfortable gym clothes have prepared many large men and women for a lifetime of inactivity. If exercise has come to mean humiliation and failure, it can be hard to break out of the vicious circle of poor fitness, non-participation and low self-esteem.

Yet there are large people who take part in sport and exercise very successfully – weightlifters, field athletes, rugby players, judo experts, swimmers, all kinds of big sportsmen and women at the highest levels. At the amateur level, many large people have overcome their reservations to take part in every conceivable form of physical activity from aerobics to gardening.

Of course, it is vital that each individual should be aware of his or her limitations. A very large person would be ill-advised to take up a strenuous sport without a thorough medical checkup. Nevertheless, with careful planning and a sensible approach, almost every large person can find some sort of healthful, enjoyable activity.

Big, beautiful and fit: Elizabeth's story

Eight years ago, when she was 27, Elizabeth decided that she had had enough of feeling that her size was her fault. A lifelong vegetarian and sensible eater, she resented the implication that she had an eating disorder. 'This is just the way that I am,' she explains. 'I looked at photographs of my great-grandmothers, and they were all like me.'

Around this time, Nancy Roberts was writing her influential book, *Breaking All the Rules*. As part of her research and preparation, she got together with a ballet dancer and teacher, Michael Manning, who sadly passed away during 1990, to create a new concept in exercise classes: 'Big, Beautiful and Fit' (BBF). Elizabeth heard about the new classes in central London, and decided to go along with two of her friends. It was a decision which changed her life.

The classes were born at the height of the 'aerobics' boom, but they didn't just consist of standard aerobic exercises. They were specially adapted by Michael Manning to suit larger bodies, taking account of the fact that many of the women who went hadn't done any exercise at all for years. Elizabeth was a case in point:

I never thought I was a particularly active person. Then I realized that if you've got big boobs it's difficult to play sport, and you can't get the clothes, etc. I had given up swimming because I felt self-conscious. You don't exercise because you feel intimidated.

But no-one felt intimidated at BBF. In the supportive atmosphere, the women realized how much they could do, and how much pleasure they could derive from dance and movement. Elizabeth recalls:

Although there was an element of aerobic exercise, it wasn't 'going for the burn'. It was 'if it hurts, stop'. There was a lot of stretching and suppleness. Later on, Michael built some yoga into the classes. People loved it. He also incorporated a lot of ballet stretches, which we adored because we were the little girls who never went to ballet. It opened up a whole new world for us, gave us a variety of different experiences.

BBF was free from competitiveness and from pressure, unlike the old school PE classes. Another source of pride was that there were never any injuries at BBF classes, because every movement had been thoroughly tried, tested and approved by medical experts. Elizabeth feels that one of the great secrets of the classes was Michael Manning's rapport with the group members.

The physical benefits of the classes were quickly apparent to Elizabeth. Although she did not lose weight, she felt immediately better:

I toned up enormously. The exercise must have increased my metabolism, and I felt much more energetic. Exercise apparently releases natural endorphins, and makes you feel better. Even if I went to a class tired, I would come out refreshed. I felt I was using my body better in everyday life, that I was becoming more supple and building up my stamina.

Yet the benefits were far greater than just firmer muscles and flexibility. Elizabeth feels that the supportive nature of the groups cannot be overestimated.

When you go to a class with other large women, suddenly you're not the only one in the world. You exchange tips – for example about clothes. You find they are very willing to share that information. You begin to think 'I'm worth something', and 'I deserve it'. Unity is strength!

So successful were the classes that there were soon too many for Michael to teach single-handed, so Elizabeth began to take some of them herself. Now she herself was providing a role-model for the large women who came to the class. 'If she can do it,' they thought, 'maybe I can, too.' From non-athlete to dance teacher in a few months, Elizabeth had come a long way.

Unfortunately, like many evening classes, Big, Beautiful and Fit has suffered from declining numbers. Classes can only be run if they are economically viable. Elizabeth's number is given at the end of this chapter, for anyone interested in joining a new class.

Exercise: why me?

Many large people make the mistake of thinking that they have to become thin before they can exercise. How wrong they are. As long as the exercise is suited to your taste, ability and general health, there is no reason why you can't have fun whatever your size. Exercise shouldn't become something you'll allow yourself to do 'when I'm thin'. You don't have to aim for a 'perfect' body, and you have the right to set your own, achievable goals. Incidentally, if your chosen activity isn't fun you should stop and try something else, because you'll never stick at something you dislike.

But why exercise?

- to improve your health: stamina, cardiovascular system, strength, suppleness
- to improve your appearance (you won't necessarily lose weight but you will improve your muscle tone)
- to improve your self-esteem: by showing your body you care you reinforce your self-esteem; also, the release of endorphins can give you a real sense of wellbeing
- to achieve goals which you have set yourself: a sense of personal achievement is a great confidence-booster
- to make social contact with others: either as part of a special group for large people (like BBF) or as a member of an 'ordinary' team or class; always standing on the sidelines excludes you from social contact and confirms the general opinion that 'fat people don't exercise'
- to rediscover pleasure in your body: once you have started to exercise, however gently, you will begin to feel how pleasurable movement can be, and how natural it is for your body to exercise. This will build up your acceptance of your body and help you to listen to its 'signals' – hunger, movement, illness etc.

What kind of exercise should I do?

The type of exercise that you choose will be determined by:

- your personality: do you prefer to exercise alone or in a group, competitively or non-competitively?
- your preferences: do you enjoy water sports, team games, dance movements, vigorous exercise etc?
- your aptitudes: is your coordination reasonably good, or are ballgames a constant embarrassment because you can never hit the ball?
- your goals: what type and degree of fitness are you aiming for? Is your main goal pleasure?
- your general level of health: it is always advisable to discuss your choice of exercise with a doctor, in case there are medical factors to consider. If in doubt, exercise with caution and stop at the first sign of distress or discomfort. Don't let others push you beyond the level of your ability.

Generally speaking, the best sort of exercise for large people is 'low-impact' activity such as swimming, which puts no strain on the joints. High-impact exercise like jogging or the traditional aerobic workout tends to overload joints: every time your foot hits the ground, your body is jarred by the extra weight. This can lead to all sorts of injuries. BBF exercises have been adapted to suit larger women – for example, in 'running on the spot', the toe never actually leaves the ground.

Another thing to avoid is lying flat on your back on the floor: as large people tend to have large bottoms, their spines do not lie flat against the ground and this puts a strain on the back. It is best to flex the knees, as this produces a nice straight back. Touching your toes is generally not recommended, either, as it also strains the body. Remember: *you* are the best judge of what feels good, but only as long as you listen to your body and don't ignore any pain signals.

Stretching and exercising to music

'Big, Beautiful and Fit' classes come into this category, and this type of exercise is very popular with people of all sizes. Exercising to music is much more fun than just doing a series of boring and repetitive exercises on the bedroom floor. If you are just starting out after a long period of inactivity, gentle stretching exercises are an ideal way to build up suppleness and discover your potential. Also, you can do this at home (to 'Top of the Pops') until you have plucked up courage to join a class! Exercise videos specifically designed for large people are available in America, though I do not know of any yet in this country.

Individual sports and activities

If you are self-conscious about your body, or simply prefer to be on your own when you are exercising, there is a wide choice of sports and exercise options. Most experts discourage large people from suddenly taking up a very strenuous activity like squash, for instance, so it is best to start off with something fairly slow, gentle and controllable. You could try walking – picking up speed and increasing the distance as you gain in stamina – or cycling (you can always use an exercise bike if you don't fancy going out on the road).

Swimming

Swimming is the best all-round exercise of all. Understandably, many large people refuse to go swimming in a public pool because of the stares and abuse they suffer. This is really quite ironic, since many of the world's top distance swimmers are very large and extremely fit. American swimmer Lynne Cox (who has broken both the male and female world records for the Channel crossing) weighs nearly 94 kg (15 stone) and owes her success to the fact that her body is around 40 per cent fat.

Some large people decide that they will get together and hire a pool for a session each week, although others say that they would rather not be 'segregated': why should they have to exercise separately from other people? Perhaps the best solution is simply to find one or two friends and go along together. Once you're in the water, who cares what shape you are anyway?

Exercising with others

Taking that first step and joining a group or a club can be a stressful moment for anyone, large or not. Exercising with others means exposing your body with all its shortcomings, and it's only too easy to imagine that everyone will spend the whole time staring at you and thinking how fat you are.

In most cases, this won't happen. They might look at you a few times at the start, but give it ten minutes and they'll have forgotten about your size, particularly if you're joining in enthusiastically. Elizabeth recommends that, if you are thinking of joining an exercise class, you should try to ask the teacher some questions before you commit yourself: What level of class is it? Are you sympathetic to large class members? Can I stand at the back to start off with? You don't have to wear a leotard, and you can make it clear that you will leave if you are singled out in any way. Best of all, go along with a few friends who can give you moral support.

Many large people enjoy playing tennis and badminton, which provide excellent opportunities for social contact and confidence-building. Perhaps the greatest fun of all is dancing. Whether it's foxtrot, lambada or simply moving about in time to the music, it's an excellent form of exercise that you can tailor to your individual needs and preferences.

Exercise in everyday life

Exercise doesn't have to mean sport. You don't have to revolutionize your way of life if you don't want to. In fact, you may already be more active than you think, particularly if you have young children.

Actress Annette Badland has her own very positive prescription for a healthy outdoor life: she enjoys walking, swimming and yoga, and also grows organic vegetables on her allotment. She finds that these activities allow her to meet people, to improve her health, and – in the case of the allotment – to express her creativity:

> I think you can be big, fit and healthy – I do my best! I swim in a public pool, though I do feel anxious about diving in. I get defiant: why should I reduce my life just to satisfy other people? I won't do it. I do yoga, which I can adapt to my own limitations. It's purely personal and involves the whole of your being. I'm also a vegetarian, and don't drink coffee or tea these days because I used to be a coffee-holic.
>
> Gardening helps me enormously. It's a very productive thing to do. I get a tremendous sense of satisfaction from watching things grow. I knew someone who weighed around 125 kg (20 stone) and told me that she couldn't garden, because she found it impossible to bend down. So I told her 'Sit on your bottom – that's what I do when I get tired'. She tried it, and it worked. I like walking, too. You can do it at your own pace, and it means you're not restricting your view of the world. You encounter other people instead of just sitting alone in your room, worrying. Good things are bound to come out of that.

Astrid's success story

If you were a regular reader of *Extra Special*, you will remember Astrid Longhurst. She was ES's 'fitness fun-atic' – a big, beautiful fitness expert whose exercise pages were illustrated with plump, smiling cartoon ladies enjoying themselves keeping fit.

Extra Special is no more, alas, but Astrid is blossoming. She has a flourishing career as a size 16–18 model; she also runs her own fitness company, and exercise classes for people of both sexes, all ages and sizes, and also designs personalized exercise programmes.

At first glance, it is easy to think that Astrid has always had all the answers. She looks so radiant and healthy that it is difficult to imagine her any other way. Yet Astrid had to overcome both bulimia nervosa and a major weight problem before she learned to live in peace with her naturally large body.

At fifteen, Astrid weighed over 94 kg (15 stone) and was a size 24. Her teachers told her to forget becoming a dancer, as she was just 'too fat'. Desperate to fulfil her ambition, she went on a diet. By the age of nineteen she weighed only 60 kg (9 stone 7 lbs) – and was accepted by a dance school. She was also runner-up in the national Slimmer of the Year contest.

But all was not well. Along with artificial slenderness came perpetual hunger and an obsession with food – leading to bulimia. Gradually, Astrid moved from constant dieting towards a more natural, balanced diet. She put on weight – but stabilized at a fit 75 kg (12 stone). She has never felt better: 'I no longer try to starve to become thin and my life is no longer put "on hold" – waiting for a skinny tomorrow. The moment is NOW. I can now live in the body I have and enjoy it.'

Astrid feels that as a fit larger woman, she has a great deal to offer her pupils: 'I understand the problems and difficulties. I am not a skinny Jane Fonda lookalike and I don't offer exercises which are near-impossible to do. I feel I offer enthusiasm, understanding, possibilities and a positive attitude towards your own body and health. Size is not a limitation.'

What makes a good exercise programme?

According to Astrid, there are several things to look out for when you are choosing an exercise teacher. The programmes that she herself designs, teaches and supervises are carefully structured for large people, following British Sports Council and RSA Certificate principles for safety, structure and adaptability.

New pupils are asked to fill in a health profile, to determine whether there is any need to adapt the exercises to accommodate any problems. Body postures are checked during exercises, to avoid injuries occurring, and pupils are given plenty of praise and encouragement. If a teacher is not qualified, or does not offer this type of personal approach, you have to ask yourself if you are placing your body in good hands.

Like Elizabeth, Astrid believes that exercise is a valuable source of physical and mental wellbeing and a sense of achievement. She describes it as 'a feeling of working *with* your body, rather than against it'. She believes that the only good exercise programme is one that is within a student's capabilities, that can be maintained without becoming boring, and that fits into his or her lifestyle. An exercise programme does not have to mean just 'doing exercises'. Subject to your health, you could vary it to include yoga, golf, gentle circuit training, walking, swimming or whatever else you fancy. 'The main thing,' as Astrid says, 'is to enjoy it.'

Too big to exercise?

For very large men and women, Astrid recommends starting with a walking programme, building gradually on variation and intensity, together with gentle stretching and strength/endurance exercises – nothing too strenuous. If you have any doubts, check first with your doctor. You might consider approaching a qualified exercise expert who can prepare a safe personal programme for you, or learning the Alexander Technique (see page 122), which concentrates on body posture and awareness rather than exercise.

Fitness begins at home . . .

If you find there is no specialist exercise class in your area, and you are reticent about joining a regular class, Astrid recommends starting with your own home exercise programme, which could involve:

- going for a walk
- marching or walking on the spot to music, starting at two minutes and building up to ten minutes over a ten-week period
- buying a 'bouncer' – a fun and safe way to exercise
- getting together with a few friends and doing gentle exercises together.

This should help you to build up your self-confidence, and you can then think about 'interviewing' some of the local exercise teachers to find out which is the best class for you.

Boys will be boys

There is no reason why large men, even those who have suffered heart attacks, should not take up exercise successfully, as long as they check with their doctors and approach it sensibly. Some men enjoy circuit training and find it within their capabilities.

On the other hand, caution is the name of the game. In Astrid's experience, men sometimes push themselves too hard. In a large man who has done no exercise for a long time, this could be dangerous. She explains:

> The problem is in getting them to start gradually and build up. One man enjoyed the class so much that he would do two in a row and about five a week. This was far too much for his build and ability, and I suggested a split training regime, working every other day at a lesser intensity. He actually made more improvement this way.

Astrid's exercises

Just to get you in the mood, and just for fun, here are a few of the exercises that Astrid has developed especially for large people. They were originally published in *Extra Special*.

Spring clean workout

These are exercises based on everyday household chores, so you don't even have to take time off from your work to exercise!

Hoover mover: While vacuum cleaning let your arms, not your legs, do most of the work. Push the cleaner back and forth with a good stretching action – arms right out then back, with the elbows coming into your sides. Keep your back straight throughout – do not hunch.

Rise and shine: Transform window-cleaning into a stretch-out exercise. Clean half with each hand and as you stretch for the high bits, think of really reaching up and out of your waist. Stand on tiptoe to reach the topmost glass keeping your legs straight – see that you don't bend the knees.

Pool your resources

These are exercises you can do in a swimming pool: you work against the resistance of the water, and it supports your weight.

Sea legs: Stand waist deep, holding the side with one hand. Raise the outside leg sideways as far as you can, then lower it. Really push against the water. Do this ten to twenty times, change sides and repeat with the other leg.

Fish tail: Face the poolside and hold the edge with both hands. Raise both knees towards the chest and let the body lean forward. Now push both legs out firmly behind you, then return them. Do this ten to twenty times.

Winter warmers

These are exercises to keep you warm and to stimulate the circulation.

Walk 'n' jog: Start by walking on the spot, then gradually increase your pace until almost jogging but don't let your toes leave the ground. Ensure you put your heels down on each step (never jog on the balls of your feet). Start with one minute a day and gradually increase to five – more if you can manage it without strain. You can do this to music –preferably something with a good beat.

Arm circles: Stand with feet shoulder-distance apart and swing your right arm in a wide circle from front to back, remembering to keep your elbow bent. Repeat without pause ten times. Then do it with the left arm, and then with both arms together.

Tea tippler

This is a relaxation exercise, for when you're sitting down at the end of the day and enjoying a cup of tea.

Sit in a comfortable chair with a cup of tea, but before you have it concentrate on your relaxation and breathing. Close your eyes; breathe in, feeling your stomach push out gently; breathe out, feeling the stomach contract gently. Just breathe normally for a few minutes, focusing your mind on your inner centre of calm. Open your eyes and sit quietly, savouring your drink.

Don't forget . . .

Before you pull on your leotard and legwarmers, here are a few points you should bear in mind. They will help to make exercise a safer and more pleasant experience:

- large people tend to get hot (fat traps heat under the skin) so you need to wear loose-fitting flexible clothing and work in a well-ventilated area. You should always warm up properly before any harder exercise, and be careful not to overdo it. A qualified instructor will know your target heart rate, and check that you don't exceed it
- body posture and alignment are very important, as people carrying extra weight often find that their body balance is out of order, putting a strain on the body. Astrid recommends sitting exercises

111

(in a chair) as a good way to begin correcting the alignment, and exercise the rest of the body safely and comfortably

- if you find lying on the floor uncomfortable, support yourself with mats or cushions
- shoes should support the feet but allow them to move unrestricted; Astrid particularly recommends Reeboks or Avia
- be aware of your general health and any limitations it might place on you. Have you had your blood pressure checked? Are you taking any medication? Have you had a recent operation or injury? How large are you? How supple are you? Don't take chances with your body
- don't ever let anyone push you beyond what is comfortable for you. *If it is painful, stop immediately*. Don't let your pride lead you into unnecessary injuries
- visit the toilet before class
- don't eat a heavy meal within two hours of exercising
- try different types of activity to find out which suit you best: you might hate exercises but love gardening or golf
- don't feel you must limit yourself to one type of activity – variety is the spice of life
- don't assume that you can't be graceful, strong, supple and skilful
- *think positive*: don't let anyone make you feel ashamed of your body.

Useful addresses

Big, Beautiful and Fit groups: contact Elizabeth Osborne (tel: 081 883 8732)

Hard Bodies Workout Company (Astrid Longhurst): (tel: 0628 21307)

In the United States, various companies offer exercise videos for large women. At the time of writing, these included:

Women in Motion . . . an odyssey (video aerobic workout for the large-sized woman), includes low-impact exercises designed in consultation with doctors; available from:

Big Tape Enterprises
PO Box 5978
Bethesda
MD 20814
USA

Women at Large 'Breakout' (exercise video); available from:
The Fitness Group
PO Box 251
Edmonds
WA 98020
USA

Further reading

Breaking All the Rules, Nancy Roberts (New York: Viking, 1985)
Great Shape: First Fitness Guide for Large Women, Pat Lyons RN and
Debby Burgard (Palo Alto, California: Bull Publishing Co., 1990)

7

A New You:
Building your Inner Image

It is possible to develop a fitter, healthier, more beautiful body – whatever your size. You owe it to yourself to stop ignoring or mistreating your body and set about making the most of it. Whether or not your lifeplan involves losing weight is entirely up to you: the keywords are health, acceptance and pleasure in your physical being.

A healthier body should make you feel better about yourself. But this may not be enough to tackle the fundamental problem of body image. The self-esteem of many large men and women is extremely low, and an unfit or neglected body can be a result of deepseated feelings of worthlessness and guilt. Even if you are physically fit, you may still provoke negative reactions from other people if you are projecting a negative inner image.

In this chapter, we ask two important questions:

● why do large people so often feel bad about themselves?
● what can you do to improve your own self-image?

The culpability trap

As I have mentioned earlier in this book, being fat is not a moral issue. But unfortunately a lot of fat people are made to feel as if it is. This is the 'culpability trap', in which feelings of guilt and worthlessness are imposed upon us. We may think that when we look at our bodies and say 'yuk' that is an objective judgement – but in fact we are simply voicing the accepted values of a society in which thin is good and beautiful and fat is bad and ugly.

Men may suffer less than women, since they are not expected to spend hours in front of a mirror, preening themselves for approval. They may also be rather less embarrassed than women about taking up 'more than their fair share' of space. Women are brought up from birth to believe that they should conform to very rigid standards of appearance and behaviour.

The plain girl is pitied, since she 'cannot help' the way she looks. The fat girl is punished, because not only is she imposing an unnecessary 'ugliness' upon herself – she is also challenging the

114

female stereotype by daring to have a large body. Since she is apparently determined to be 'ugly' and therefore 'undesirable', she is also challenging the accepted doctrine that women shall attract men who will then take over the responsibility for their lives.

Being big from childhood means a lifetime of being told you are 'not good enough', that you are 'defective' and that you will only earn approval when you learn to conform (that is, lose weight). Parental criticism early in life can instil deep feelings of anxiety and guilt. Some children grow up to become obsessive perfectionists, unable to derive satisfaction from any success (however dazzling) because they suspect that they could perhaps have worked a little harder, given 110 per cent instead of just 100 per cent.

It is not difficult to see how a fat child can grow up feeling like a second-class citizen if he or she has bad experiences in childhood. Fat adults can feel just as bad because the whole of society seems against them. Some feel so worthless that they live with partners who abuse them for their size ('I'm so fat, I don't deserve a good relationship – I should be glad that anyone's prepared to live with me, looking like this'); and accumulate 'friends' who lower their self-esteem with catty remarks.

Isolation and poor self-esteem very often leads to a complete lack of assertiveness, as psychologist Susan Howard explains:

> Acknowledging that she has rights at all can be a major undertaking for the large woman. This is because many (though not all) of them lack the self-confidence of self-esteem to believe it. . . . This originates from the tendency of girls to base their self-esteem on how others evaluate them. . . . Since it is normal in our society for people to devalue fat people (and for fat people to do the same) it is doubly difficult for the fat woman to value herself. And if you have little confidence in yourself it becomes hard to believe you have any rights at all ('The right to be large', part 2, *Extra Special*).

Society's implication is that fat people have forfeited their right to have relationships, to be treated with respect, to have normal feelings and opinions and – above all – to express them. Being assertive means changing from within to challenge prejudice – but the good news is that self-assertion can help large people to achieve the equality which is theirs by right.

The level of a person's inner self-esteem is usually reflected in external ways. A large person may express his or her dissatisfaction and lack of confidence through all, or some, of the following.

115

Clothes

Many fat people use their clothes as 'camouflage' for bodies they are ashamed of. Ann Harper, a famous American 'queen-size' model, relates the story of her friend Vicki who thought of herself as a 'beautiful floating head'. She behaved as though her body didn't exist, because she hated it so much. So although her hair and make up were always immaculate, her body was perpetually hidden in a shapeless, black sack-dress. It was as though she lived only from the neck up (Harper and Lewis, *The Big Beauty Book*).

Other large women tackle the problem differently. They know that their bodies exist, and that they are 'defective', but they refuse to accept them as they are. Some pretend that squeezing their size 22 bodies into size 14 clothes turns them into size 14 ladies. Others – perhaps a modest size 16 – buy everything two sizes too big because they believe that people will think they are thin and insubstantial if their clothes are hanging off them! Either way, the effect is disastrous because only clothes that fit well look good. People are perfectly aware of your size, so it's pointless trying to hide it.

General appearance and grooming: self-neglect

A large person who is trying to ignore his or her body will probably refuse to take any notice of its needs. This can lead to a scruffy, unkempt, neglected appearance. People who imagine they are only fat 'temporarily', or who feel that their size is 'shameful', may deprive themselves of a lot of pleasure by refusing to spend money on themselves. 'What's the point?' they say. 'No matter how much I dress up, people will still laugh at me. I'll wait until I'm thin, and then I'll spoil myself.' But if they never are thin, think of the deprivation they'll have suffered.

Body language

It has been estimated that 70–90 per cent of all communication messages are conveyed through non-verbal signals, such as body language. A person who is ashamed of his or her body will convey that negativity to those around – for example, by hunching the shoulders, avoiding eye contact. Changing the signals you send out can alter the way in which other people react to you.

Tone of voice

Like body language, the tone and inflection of the voice convey a multitude of signals to those around you. You can become aware of the way you speak and change it to positive effect.

Withdrawal from social contact

Some fat people believe that if they withdraw from competition and contact with others, they will avoid stressful situations in which they feel inferior. Unfortunately, they also miss out on most of the pleasures of life. As we have seen, sport is one area from which fat people often feel they must exclude themselves in order to avoid ridicule. But why should they? Confidence-building techniques can help you cope with any prejudice and may help to reduce it because of the positive messages that you will send out about your body.

Passivity and 'people pleasing'

Are you a doormat? Many large people are, because they feel anxious or scared about doing anything which might cause other people to criticize them. Many a large lady has earned herself compliments for her 'reliability' or her 'caring attitude' and 'ready smile'. She is the one who's always ready to babysit at the last minute, or to listen to everyone else's problems even if she doesn't find them very interesting.

Who listens to hers? Probably no-one. Fat people aren't supposed to have problems. 'Nice' fat people are supposed to be jolly and obliging – full of sympathy and understanding even when no-one has any sympathy for them. The only way out is to learn to say 'no' and stop being afraid of showing your own anger occasionally. Bottling up your feelings only builds up your anger and frustration.

Aggressive behaviour

At the other end of the scale is the large person who overcompensates by becoming aggressive and overbearing. This is no better than being passive, and no less stressful.

Self-deprecating remarks

We've all made jokes against ourselves from time to time, but with some large people it becomes a habit. The reason seems to be that, subconsciously, they think 'any minute now, someone is going to criticize me for being fat and stupid' – so they decide to 'get in first' by actually saying 'I'm so fat and stupid!'. If they criticize themselves, perhaps that will stop other people criticizing them? In practice, it simply undermines the respect of those around them who feel they have *carte blanche* to say anything they like. Much 'fat humour' is based on this idea.

All of the above are ways of sending negative messages to the rest of the world: 'I'm not worth bothering with'; 'I don't value myself, so why should you?' and so on. In order to provoke more positive reactions in others, you must first learn to accept yourself, to stop being your own harshest critic and dare the world not to respect you.

How do you feel about yourself?

The way you feel about your body is influenced by the society in which you live, and the views of the people around you: parents, friends, lovers – not to mention TV and the press. But that's no reason to accept all the messages that are directed at you, without question. It is *your* body, and nobody has the right to tell you how you should feel about it. It's for you to decide what it will look like. There are no 'good' bodies and 'bad' bodies, and there is no reason for you to feel unhappy with the one you have. As Eleanor Roosevelt once said, 'No-one can make you feel inferior without your consent.'

Now is the time to take control of your own body, and the way you feel about it. But before you can begin to make changes in the way you approach life, you need to look closely at:

- your feelings about yourself
- subjects and situations that make you unhappy or uncomfortable
- the image you present to the world
- other people's reactions to you
- your behaviour towards other people.

This section deals with some of the techniques and strategies you could try to help you feel more 'at ease' with your body. They can help you to get to know it; to stop pretending it doesn't exist or hating it because it seems 'unacceptable'; and to allow yourself to enjoy it just the way it is.

In some cases, readjusting your body image can be a painful experience, as it may involve going over feelings and events which have caused you distress in the past. Some people find it helpful to get together with a close friend or a support group, so that experiences and problems can be shared.

But don't be depressed if self-help techniques don't revolutionize your life; they aren't an instant panacea, and they are not going to be helpful for everybody. In many cases, their most important function will be to make you think about any problems you may have, and accept that you need help in order to resolve them. You may eventually choose to consult a professional therapist or counsellor, who can make informed suggestions about the best programme for you. A list of contact addresses is given at the end of this chapter.

Whatever you decide to do – even if it is to do nothing – it is vital to remember that you are *all right as you are*. If you can accept that and live your life accordingly, others will follow.

Picture this . . .

Visualization is a technique which you may have heard about in connection with the treatment of cancer. After lengthy trials and much scepticism, doctors have at last been forced to admit that the mind can be a powerful tool for healing.

In this type of physical healing, sufferers are taught to visualize their white blood cells as golden bullets, attacking the malignant cancer cells. This process really works – though no-one is quite sure how.

You may be wondering what this has to do with your body image. But creative visualization has been used for many years by therapists working with women – some of them sufferers from eating disorders, some not – to help them search inside themselves and put right the causes of their poor body image.

As with cancer therapy, the principle is the acceptance of the mind's enormous power to change and to heal. If the influence of other people can change the way you feel about yourself, how much greater is your own mind's power to influence your self-image?

Imagination can be used to practise new attitudes and behaviour patterns. When we use our imagination, something psychologically real happens. As far as our minds are concerned, we are living whatever we are imagining. Take the example of professional musicians and skilled craftspeople. Many of them have come to recognize that they can improve their technique simply by using imagination to go over and over the different skills they use, again and again. They find that when they actually come to practise these skills, their technique has improved – even though they had only 'rehearsed' the skills imaginatively. Imagination really can change behaviour.

You can do this, too. By creatively visualizing yourself as behaving in a different way, or feeling differently about yourself, you can achieve that change. The only thing holding you back is the prison you have created for yourself: your own negative self-image. This, too, is a product of your imaginative powers. Think how much better it would be if you could make your imagination your ally instead of your enemy.

Discovering your body image

Through relaxation, you can explore and discover:

- how you feel in your body
- how you would like to feel
- what you want to achieve.

Remember: what you are setting out to do is to change the way you feel about yourself, not your physical appearance. This isn't just another diet and exercise programme, but an exercise programme for the mind, rather than the body.

While relaxed and lying on the floor, try 'scanning' your body to discover how aware you really are of its shape and form. Research has shown that men are generally better at estimating the size and objective appearance of their bodies, while women very often overestimate their size. The extreme example of this would be anorexia nervosa: sufferers frequently see themselves as grossly fat when they are in fact dangerously thin.

Try this exercise, and see how accurate you are:

Lie on the floor and relax, eyes gently closed. In your imagination, sense how wide your hips are. Hold your hands just over your hips, with the gap between them representing the estimated width of your hips. Lower them until they are on a level with your hips. Open your eyes, and check whether you were right or not. Are you surprised by your accuracy or inaccuracy? If your mental estimate was very inaccurate, maybe you don't know your body as well as you thought you did. Try the same exercise with different parts of your body –your head, thighs etc – and find out which you 'know' best.

You might also like to try another exercise in which you visualize yourself standing in front of a mirror – first fully clothed, and then naked. The idea is to explore the way you 'look' at yourself in the mirror each time: are your reactions different when you are naked? Are there any parts of your body that particularly please you, or that you are ashamed of? Does your posture change when you imagine yourself naked? (for example, are you hunched up, or trying to hide your body from yourself?)

The above exercises are useful in helping you to develop a clearer, more realistic picture of your body – particularly if you tend to think of yourself as a 'beautiful floating head', and avoid thinking about your body at all.

Influences and confrontations

If you have a poor self-image, the chances are that it has its roots way back in your childhood and adolescence. Visualization can be used to help you go back in time and recreate imaginatively your growth, the turning-points and confrontations in your life.

You may choose to imagine yourself face to face with some of the influential adults who shaped you as a person, exploring the way you feel in their presence and perhaps communicating some of the anger, frustration or love you have never been able to put into words.

Another useful exercise is to imagine yourself surrounded by a circle of all those people who have contributed to your negative view of your own beauty. Turning in your mind's eye to each one in turn, you express what you feel and give each person a chance to respond. You can then decide whether or not you wish to forgive each person and, if so, free yourself from the bonds of negative emotion which bind you to him or her.

Forgiveness is a healing experience, but it is also a difficult one. If you have spent many years full of hatred, anger or pain, it will probably take time and patience to free yourself – but it will be worth it.

Calling a truce with the mirror

Just because you are large, you should not feel you must punish yourself by depriving yourself of an active, healthy, happy existence. Large people often subconsciously punish their bodies or ignore them because they are not 'perfect'. But life doesn't wait to start until you are thin: it has already started without you! Don't let your poor body image prevent you from fulfilling your potential.

One telltale sign of a poor self-image is the inability to look calmly at your reflection in a mirror. In fact, some people banish mirrors from their homes altogether, and try to pretend that their bodies do not exist. Pretending that you are thin will not *make* you thin. But accepting that you are big and physically attractive may do wonders for the way in which others perceive you. Sooner or later, you will accept the positive messages that you are sending to yourself, and become truly confident.

One useful exercise in accepting your body involves sitting in front of a full-length mirror. First of all, you close your eyes and strike a pose which expresses the way you feel about yourself. You then strike other poses which express a series of moods (confidence, joy, withdrawal, apprehension, etc) and feel how your body moves and changes.

Still with your eyes closed, you imagine that you are now your 'ideal' size, and strike the same series of poses – noticing any difference. You may find, for example, that you carry yourself more confidently and more openly when you imagine that you are at your 'ideal' size. Why not try to emulate that same confidence as you really are, in your daily life?

Finally, you open your eyes and repeat the routine – striking poses as your real and 'ideal' selves. One of the objects of this exercise is to help you assess your body posture and body language, and adapt them for better health and a more positive image. Bad posture is not only a way of telling the world that you are ashamed of your body: it can also be unhealthy. An unbalanced skeleton can lead to muscle problems, headaches and even breathing difficulties. So if only for your health, you should think about teaching yourself to 'walk tall' and project a sense of pride in your body.

Getting started

The best way to learn visualization techniques is to attend a class. If no classes exist in your area, why not get together with a few friends and work systematically through a book of exercises? You can offer each other support, exchange experiences and keep track of your progress as you go along.

One excellent book is Dr Marcia Germaine Hutchinson's *Transforming Body Image*. This contains a ten-week programme of exercises which have been extensively tried and tested in America. Susie Orbach's *Fat is a Feminist Issue 2* also contains a number of useful exercises. Full details of resources are given at the end of this chapter.

Other ways to discover your body

Visualization is not the only way to explore your body and your own image of it. There is no method to suit everyone, so you may need to sample a few different options. Possibilities include the following.

Alexander technique

This teaches 'relaxation in activity' to make students more aware of balance, posture and movement. You are taught to 'listen' to your body's natural postural reflexes and escape from chronic muscle tensions and patterns of distortion which can result from the stresses and strains of life (including the social pressures involved in being large). Rediscovering a proper relationship with gravity enables the body's processes of movement, breathing, digestion and circulation to be carried out more effectively. Teachers of the technique use manual guidance as well as verbal instruction. This degree of physical contact can be helpful for large people who have felt for a long time that their bodies do not 'deserve' to be touched and cared for. You will probably need from 20 to 30 lessons, spread over a three to five month period. Cost varies, but at time of writing was around £6–£15 per session.

Relaxation and hypnosis

Most local colleges now offer day and evening relaxation courses, at relatively little cost. Once you have learned the basic techniques involved, you can continue to use them on your own, at home or even at work. Relaxation/self-hypnosis tapes can be purchased in many health food and bookshops, though these will vary in quality and may not suit everyone. Deep relaxation not only helps you to get in touch with your body: it also improves the quality of your breathing and reduces stress. If you decide to consult a professional hypnotherapist, make sure that he or she is properly qualified, and if possible choose one by personal recommendation.

Yoga and meditation

Like relaxation, these skills are often available through local colleges and are very helpful for anyone who is seeking a more tranquil relationship between mind and body. They require the aid of a qualified teacher. Yoga is an extremely valuable form of stretching exercise for large people, as long as it is taught properly and adapted to the needs of a large body.

Deportment

Most people laugh nowadays when they hear the word 'deportment', as it is so reminiscent of well-bred Victorian ladies gliding around with books balanced on their heads! But really all it means is training for good posture and graceful movement. It is taught by many modelling schools, and a group of you might approach one of their teachers to run a special course for you.

Dance

This is not only an excellent exercise, but a wonderful way to take pleasure in your body's movement and expression. Moving to music is one of the most natural instincts in the world, so allow yourself the pleasure of self-expression and self-discovery.

Taking stock of your self-esteem

Now that you have begun to acknowledge your body's existence and needs, you can move on to assess the level of your self-esteem. This simply means discovering the value which you place upon yourself as a human being.

One way to do this is to draw up your own personal profile: a list of your positive and negative feelings about various different aspects of your life. Let us take an example: 'Sarah' is a middle-aged housewife, and a large lady. Here are some of the things she might say about herself:

Looks	Positive feelings: casual, simple Negative feelings: shapeless, dull colours, poor quality clothes
Manner	Positive feelings: warm Negative feelings: superficially cheerful
Work	Positive feelings: conscientious, a fund of good ideas Negative feelings: unassertive, afraid of criticism
Home life	Positive feelings: helpful, tidy Negative feelings: doormat, obsessive
Relationships	Positive feelings: loyal, loving Negative feelings: victim, 'mother confessor' figure, often seen as asexual
Social life	Positive feelings: supportive Negative feelings: unexciting, limited

Although it is useful to take stock of your good points (and bear them in mind at all times!) the important list to look at for the moment is the 'negative' list. Sarah has been very critical of herself, and this is not very constructive. What she needs to do now is to examine each aspect of her life and decide:

- what, specifically, she is saying about herself
- what she perceives to be her 'problem' areas
- how she could work to change the way she feels (it may mean just

learning to live with herself the way she is, or it could involve taking practical steps to reorganize her lifestyle).

Sarah talks about her looks in very negative terms: 'shapeless, dull colours, poor quality clothes'. She is saying 'I don't like my body'. She may also be saying that she wears dull, poor-quality clothing to camouflage it or punish herself. Alternatively, she may dress badly because she does not have access to the colourful clothes she would enjoy. Either way, she needs to:

- learn to accept her body
- determine that she will exercise her right to dress colourfully and well if she wants to.

Sarah sees her manner as 'superficially cheerful'. She is too obliging, too ready with the cheery smile and never with a frown on her face. More than likely, her friends and colleagues don't know that she is often sad inside; they think she is cheerful because she is 'fat and jolly' – a person without problems. Sarah needs to accept that she has a right to have both negative and positive feelings, and to express what she truly feels.

At work, Sarah is terrified of criticism – so she has become a workhorse, a perfectionist. She never says what she thinks (even though she may have a valid opinion to put forward) because she is afraid that someone will criticize her in return. She is continually conscious of her body's 'defectiveness'. If she keeps quiet and works hard, maybe no-one will notice how big and unattractive she is? Sarah must work to:

- accept that she is equal to everyone else
- assess the value of her opinions and express them when appropriate
- refuse to be treated any less well than any other employee.

At home, Sarah continues her obsessive perfectionism, believing that being ultra-tidy – the perfect housewife – she will make up in some small way for being a physical failure. Sarah is the type of wife and mother who stays up till 3 am ironing underpants, and cleans up uncomplainingly after her teenage son's disastrous all-night party. She has to learn that others will value her more if she learns to say 'no' from time to time.

Sarah's relationships are based on the fear that she will lose her lovers and her friends if she demands the same as a thin person would demand. She never criticizes in case she drives them away. She accepts a poor sex-life as inevitable because she is 'undesirable' and lucky to have a partner at all. She is always there to provide a shoulder for her thin friends (and their husbands) to cry on – always the 'big sister', never the 'sexual threat'. Sarah must see that she need not be the victim in her relationships; that friends who demand that she should subdue her own personality and live only to serve their needs are not really friends at all.

Finally, Sarah should also look at the way in which she regards her social life. She has the support of one or two good friends – maybe the odd cosy evening chatting round the fire. But if she is honest with herself, she really wants a bit of excitement in her life. She doesn't go out much socially because she's afraid people will laugh at her, not because she really does prefer a slide show at the village hall. 'Thin people's activities' will remain just that as long as fat people let them.

Drawing up your personal profile is a useful complement to the work which you have done through visualization or whatever technique you have chosen to help you get to know your body image. By now you should have a fairly good idea of how you see yourself, and the areas that you might wish to work on in order to increase your self-esteem. In the next sections, we look at ways of acknowledging and expressing your rights and needs, and presenting yourself to the world in a new, more positive way.

Taking charge

Many large people find that they have a problem with assertiveness. Some – like Sarah in the previous section – find it difficult to express what they want or need, because their self-esteem is so low. Others overcompensate for their anxieties by becoming aggressive and overbearing. In this section we shall discuss:

- techniques for improving your body image and self-esteem
- acknowledging your own needs and rights
- expressing yourself assertively
- appraising your body language/nonverbal signals
- building confidence in social situations.

Building self-esteem: affirmations

Remember: you do not have to be perfect to have good self-esteem. One way of improving your own self-image is to use a technique known as 'affirmation'.

126

Affirmations are often used in conjunction with creative visualization, to reinforce the changes that you are trying to make to the way you see yourself. They are brief, positive statements that you repeat to yourself several times a day. They represent qualities and attitudes that you would like to have, and through the process of repetition they can become psychological truths.

It is best to start with one statement. Once you have proved to yourself that the process can work, you can devise another statement, and so on. There is a special way to construct them, for example:

I, Jane, am a beautiful and intelligent woman
I, Mary, am proud of my sexuality
I, Anne, like myself and feel comfortable in my body
I, Mark, am capable of expressing my needs and opinions.

By including your own name in the affirmation, you are reinforcing the strength of its appeal to your subconscious. You can also practise your affirmations in front of a mirror, looking into your own eyes. If you find it difficult or uncomfortable at first, why not write down your affirmations instead of speaking them?

You should spend around fifteen minutes each day on your affirmations. Monitor any improvements in your own feelings, and in the reactions of those around you. Is your behaviour changing? Do you feel more comfortable or more confident?

Assertiveness: acknowledging your needs and rights

Every human being has needs and rights, which form the basis of most assertiveness training courses. If you are going to behave assertively –to 'stand up for yourself' in an honest and straightforward manner – you must first understand about the basic rights that all people have and that should always be respected. Many large people forget that they have these equal rights, and allow other people to violate them. Your list of rights will depend on your personal circumstances, but might include the following:

- the right to be treated with respect, as an equal
- the right to express my feelings
- the right to express my opinions and values
- the right to say yes or no for myself
- the right to make mistakes
- the right to change my mind
- the right to say 'I don't understand' (and ask for more information)

- the right to ask for what I want
- the right to decline responsibility for other people's problems
- the right not to depend on other people's approval
- the right to accept genuine compliments
- the right to accept valid criticism
- the right to reject invalid criticism
- the right to change
- the right not to change
- the right to succeed
- the right to fail
- the right to be alone.

Acknowledging your rights can be hard to do if you are used to running your life to please other people. Yet it is essential if you are to feel good about yourself. As assertiveness expert Beverley Hare puts it, 'treat yourself the way you would treat someone you loved very much'.

This doesn't mean that we all have a licence to be rude and selfish – to look after our own rights at the expense of other people's. The first rule of assertiveness is that assertive behaviour respects the rights of all concerned.

Psychologists have identified three main types of behaviour:

- aggressive
- passive
- assertive

As we have seen, large people are often passive but may also become aggressive. *Passive behaviour* involves ignoring one's own rights, and can lead to loss of self-respect, low self-image, pent-up anger and frustration (which is very stressful and unhealthy) and adverse reactions from those around you. Psychologists describe this type of behaviour in the phrase 'You're all right, I'm not'. In other words, the passive person behaves as though he or she is constantly inferior or in the wrong.

Passive people tend to avoid confrontations and daren't risk anger because they feel they will provoke too much hostility in the other, 'better and stronger', person. They take it on the nose, probably laugh it all off, and then go home and cry. That is why many large people take so much abuse and discrimination without complaint: they have been brainwashed into thinking they are inferior and don't deserve to show their feelings or be treated respectfully.

Aggressive behaviour involves steamrollering everyone else's rights and being entirely insensitive. It may get you what you want in the short term, but ultimately causes more problems than it solves. Manipulative behaviour is also a type of aggression – in which 'sneaky' behaviour is used to gain a result which still negates the other person's rights, although it may avoid the confrontation that is characteristic of overt aggressive behaviour. In aggressive behaviour, the attitude is one of 'I'm all right, you're not' – in other words, 'I'm right and if you disagree with me you must be stupid'.

The essence of *assertive behaviour* is a balanced and sensitive approach: 'I'm all right, and so are you'. To put it another way, 'I'm prepared to listen to your point of view if you're prepared to listen to mine. If we can't come to an immediate agreement, we'll find a compromise.'

Straightforwardness, honesty and give-and-take are all important elements. You state your needs, your opinions, your feelings or your values directly and without malice. You don't avoid anger, but you don't lose your temper and become aggressive. While no-one is perfect (we all blow our top or back down from time to time) assertiveness is the best form of behaviour to aim at; it is dignified, reduces frustration and anger, and enables you to provoke positive reactions in other people. It is very difficult not to respect someone who behaves assertively.

Evaluating your own behaviour

Just for fun, read through these problem situations, and decide how you would behave. Your responses indicate whether you would favour passive, aggressive or assertive behaviour.

1   The girl next door insists on playing loud music at all hours of the day and night, when you are trying to sleep. What do you do?

(a) say nothing and hope it goes away
(b) bang on the wall, shout abuse and turn your own music up
(c) call round and ask her to keep the volume low in future.

2   At work, you supervise a trainee who has been late every day for a week. What do you do?

(a) shout at him and tell him he's lazy
(b) grumble about him to all your colleagues but say nothing to him
(c) ask him if he has a reason, as you have a right to know.

3   You come home after a hard day at work, to find that your flatmate has left the place in a terrible mess. What do you do?

(a) clear it up without complaint
(b) tell him/her it really isn't fair to leave a mess, and ask him/her to clear it up
(c) make a scene.

4   Your brand-new toaster breaks down the first time you use it. What do you do?

(a) sigh, throw it away and forget about it
(b) take the remains of the toaster back to the shop with the receipt, and ask for a refund
(c) have an angry confrontation with the manager and threaten to complain to Esther Rantzen.

How did you fare? Check your answers:

Passive: 1a, 2b, 3a, 4a
Aggressive: 1b, 2a, 3c, 4c
Assertive: 1c, 2c, 3b, 4b

Taking the first step

Behaving assertively is a very important part of good self-esteem. Sorting out a problem situation assertively will always make you feel better, even if the ultimate solution isn't exactly the one you would have chosen.

If you have a problem with self-assertion – and many large people do – then without a doubt the best thing to do is to take a formal self-assertion course, organized by qualified and experienced trainers. If you know other large men and/or women in your area, you might consider getting together to put on your own assertiveness course. Your local library or women's centre will probably have details of assertiveness courses and teachers, and other useful addresses are given at the end of this chapter.

A good adjunct to assertiveness training is counselling or – even better – co-counselling. Co-counselling is a self-help therapy in which you and another individual are taught counselling techniques so that you can counsel each other. This is particularly useful for anyone who lacks close friends or who finds it difficult to express feelings to strangers.

While you are waiting to start your course, why not take your first steps towards assertiveness? You don't have to be a doormat! Here are just a few of the areas you might like to work on.

People-pleasing   Your self-esteem mustn't depend on the good opinions of others. If it does, that means that you are living your life for someone else – besides which, sooner or later you are bound to upset someone and it will all have been in vain. Try to start valuing yourself and your own judgement. Risk disapproval and anger – the consequences may not be as disastrous as you think!

Accepting negative feelings   Your body size has nothing to do with your personality, and you certainly don't have to fit into any 'fat and jolly' stereotype. If you have negative feelings like anger, these have a right to be expressed along with your positive feelings.

Bad relationships   Being fat does not affect your entitlement to good relationships. If friends or lovers are abusing you and making you feel worthless and guilty, maybe it's time to question the basis of the relationship.

Running yourself down   Stop criticizing yourself and accept that you deserve respect. Stop apologizing for your size. If you tell people 'I'm so fat and stupid', they're going to end up believing you.

The inescapable 'yes'   Learn to say 'no' occasionally, and refuse to put yourself last. When your favours are granted more sparingly, people will stop taking you for granted. It's one thing being reliable, but people won't respect you for being a doormat.

Confrontation time   Members of support groups always make a point of confronting injustice, discrimination and prejudice. It is a difficult thing to do, but if someone makes a jibe at you in the street, it really is much better to confront that person, rather than bow your head and scuttle away to cry in a corner. Most people are profoundly embarrassed if you go up to them and say, quite calmly, 'Perhaps you'd like to say something to my face?' Ignorance is the basis of most insults. Once large people show themselves to be real people, with feelings and personalities, it is a great deal harder to insult them as comic caricatures.

Compliments and criticism   Don't be one of those large people who accept all criticism as valid and all compliments as lies. If someone criticizes you for a bad mistake, it's all right to admit it: 'Yes, you're right. I did make a mistake but it won't happen again.' There's no need to grovel or to get angry. But if you know the criticism is unjustified, then you must say so, directly and firmly: 'No, that's not true. I'm not always late for work. In fact, more often than not I'm early.'

Equally, don't let your habitually low self-esteem convince you that every compliment is a sarcastic jibe or thinly disguised insult. If someone says 'You look beautiful tonight', or 'That's a nice outfit you're wearing' – and you know in your heart that it's true – then accept the compliment. Don't laugh it off: just say 'Thank you' and enjoy it.

Body language: getting your message across

All too often, we forget that 70–90 per cent of all communication messages between people are non-verbal: through gestures, expressions, tone of voice etc. In order to achieve effective assertive behaviour, it's important to ask yourself if you are sending out the right signals. If you are smiling apologetically, it will be difficult for you to tell someone you are very angry. If you are shuffling your feet and staring at the ground, how can you put across your point of view authoritatively?

The key is to harmonize the content of what you are saying with the way in which you are saying it. If the two are contradictory, the message becomes confused. Here are some of the factors to bear in mind:

- tone of voice
- inflection
- speed of speech
- eye contact
- body posture
- hand gestures
- facial expressions.

If you are *passive*, you will tend to avoid direct eye contact – looking away or down. You may smile at inappropriate moments (for example, when you ought to look firm, or angry). You may fidget uncomfortably, shuffling your feet or wringing your hands. Many passive people hunch or slump their shoulders – also a characteristic of many fat and tall people who feel ashamed of taking up space. The passive person may talk in a whining tone, or in a voice which is soft and difficult to hear. Non-assertive people are often fond of 'non-words' – like 'you know' and 'OK' – which detract from the power of what they are saying. Sometimes they turn a statement into a question, by saying 'don't you think?'

The *aggressive* speaker turns every encounter into a battle. Eye contact is direct and rather ferocious, though aggressive people may also appear bored. They sometimes stand with their hands on their hips, or jab at the other person with an accusing finger, closing in on their 'adversaries' and invading their personal space. They may talk loudly or in a deathly soft and cold voice, and often resort to sarcasm.

What you are aiming at is an *assertive* image. Assertive speakers are confident enough to maintain direct, natural eye contact, but don't resort to the aggressive speaker's 'battle tactics'. The body is relaxed and upright, and gestures open. Hand gestures are used, but only to emphasize words. The tone of voice is firm or warm, as appropriate in the situation, and the assertive speaker never invades the other person's personal space.

Please yourself!

In the final reckoning, you are the only person who *has* to live with you, 24 hours a day for your entire life. Anyone with any common-sense can see that this makes your wishes for your own self-development far more important than anyone else's. We all have to have give and take, of course, but it's no good living your life simply to please somebody else if it doesn't also please you. The following sections are about developing your own personal style and planning for the rest of your life.

Out and about: building confidence in social situations

If you are going to feel and behave more positively, you'll probably need some help from other people. It's hard to do it all on your own. You may also decide to augment an assertion course or visualization classes with other social activities which help you to build your confidence, learn new skills and acquire interesting new topics of conversation. Why not consider one or more of the following?

- joining or forming a support group: apart from the social support which this can offer, many groups get involved in practical projects such as maintaining directories of tried and tested shops, theatres etc in the area
- getting involved in your local community: voluntary work, clubs and societies and local politics are all out there, just waiting to hear from big, motivated people who want to show how much they have to offer. You could even follow the lead of the Spare Tyre Theatre Group, and get involved in size-related drama – a therapeutic and educational experience
- learning a new skill: joining an adult education class can be a turning point for many people. You have the experience of being

an accepted member of a group, added to which you have the satisfaction of week-by-week goals and achievements. Whether it's pottery or public speaking, it will probably lead on to greater things. There is no need to be isolated if you don't want to be.

Be kind to yourself

Whatever size or shape you are, you're probably your own worst critic. Learning to assert yourself and accept the body you have can be like coming out from under an enormous black cloud. Suddenly you realize that for years you have been depriving yourself of all sorts of pleasures, simply because other people thought you didn't deserve them. Now is the time to catch up on everything you've been missing!

Nancy Roberts's excellent book *Breaking All The Rules* is a good starting-point for anyone who wants a complete new image in terms of clothes, hair and makeup, but needs some practical advice. We may not all have it in us to be as daring or extravagant as Ms Roberts, but we can learn a lot from her adventurous approach. Your library should be able to get a copy for you.

Clothes in traditional 'outsize' outlets like Evans may sometimes be depressing and conventional, but there are opportunities to be different if you're prepared to spend time and imagination looking. Admittedly, it's infuriating to see a beautiful dress which would suit you to a T but which only goes up to a size 14 (why, oh why, do they do it?), but if you can swallow your resentment and go shopping with determination, there are still sartorial adventures to be had. Men's clothes, charity shops and period clothing specialists, dressmakers and generously cut 'ordinary-sized' clothes all offer additions to the limited large-size fashions currently available at reasonable prices. Catalogues, too, are beginning to provide better-quality clothing at reasonable prices.

Dale Goday's book *Dressing Thin* is rather out of favour nowadays, as most large people know very well that there's not much point in hoping that vertical stripes or a V-neck are going to transform a size 24 into the image of a size 12. But Ms Goday does understand that a large woman can also be a beautiful woman, and that other people's reactions to us are influenced not only by what we wear, but by the way we feel inside:

Lillian (Russell) didn't have a 'weight problem'. She just had weight. She knew how to be big *and* beautiful. *Her* signal to the world was loud and clear: 'I am a beauty. I dress like one. I move like one. I feel like one. Everything about me is beautiful. Men adore me, and why not? They care about me because I care about myself. You can see that just by looking at me.'

The rules – as Ms Roberts so emphatically states – are there to be broken. You don't have to avoid horizontal stripes just because they'll 'make you look fatter'. Everyone knows how big you are, anyway. Do you really think that a few stripes will make much difference? What matters is how you wear those stripes. Do they make you feel good? If not, don't wear them. If so, forget what the world says – if you feel great, you'll probably radiate confidence and look terrific.

Three important things to look for in clothes are:

- comfort: if something is badly cut or itchy, you will wriggle about and look ill at ease. It doesn't matter what size you are: you have the right to enjoy comfortable clothing
- taste: that special element which turns an ordinary outfit into a classy one
- fit: don't let pride get the better of you. If you're between sizes, buy the larger one. Don't buy anything too tight or too voluminous. Don't be fobbed off with second best and don't be pressurized by bossy assistants unless *you* know that it fits and suits you.

If clothes shops and manufacturers don't give you what you want, write to them and tell them so. Phone them up and complain. Better still, get all the large people you know to turn up on their doorstep. If enough people make a noise, they won't be able to ignore the demand any longer. Why should *you* have to take sewing lessons, when your thin friend walks into any chain store and buys something off the peg? Don't give in, and don't allow yourself to neglect your appearance because that will destroy your self-esteem.

Pampering yourself is not just for the thin people. Enjoy your body and reassure it that it is appreciated. It works hard every day, and it deserves the best. Every scented bath, every foot massage you give it will reinforce your acceptance of your body as it is. There are so many things to do to give yourself pleasure:

- have a massage or a sauna
- have a reflexology treatment
- try aromatherapy

- host a dinner party and cook beautiful gourmet food
- dress up and go out on the town
- get together with other large people and have a night out at the local disco
- buy an outfit
- spend time reading or visiting a museum
- spend money on your personal development
- learn a new craft or creative hobby like gardening
- take a modelling course and put on a large-size fashion show
- have a professional manicure or facial
- treat yourself to exotic lingerie in sumptuous fabrics.

Beating the blues

Although this book is about adopting a positive attitude to your size, it would be foolish to pretend that we can all feel good, all the time. There will always be days when the world looks black and you wonder how you could ever think good things about yourself. On those days, why not try one of these 'gloombusters'?

Intensive negativity   You might think this is the last thing you need when you're depressed, but in short bursts it can work wonders. Think your blackest, gloomiest, most murderous thoughts (and nothing else) for five minutes and five minutes only. Then make yourself switch off and think about something else. This is a good way to avoid the awful 'snowball' effect of continuously worrying about something that gets bigger and bigger until you're almost hysterical.

Going for the burn   Not – as you might imagine – an aerobics session, but a clever psychological ploy. Get a piece of paper (several if you're really down!) and write down everything you feel. You must include every thought, no matter how ashamed or guilty it makes you feel. No-one else will see it. Then tear it up into tiny pieces, and burn it. Now you can start your life afresh.

Life doesn't have to be bad because you are large. In fact, it can be extremely good. Changing other people's attitudes is an important part of it, but the process has to start within yourself. Ultimately, other people will accept the image of yourself which you 'sell' to them. It's up to you to try to make it a positive one.

Develop your own style, your own image, and don't be afraid to be different, if that's what pleases you. Some of the most confident and fulfilled large people are the most dramatic. Above all, vow never to let your size prevent you from doing anything you really want to do – whether it's a trip to Sainsbury's or a hot air balloon-flight over the Grand Canyon.

Useful addresses

Society of Teachers of the Alexander Technique
10 London House
266 Fulham Road
London SW10 9EL (send SAE for list of names and addresses of teachers who have graduated from an approved three-year training programme)

Meditation, relaxation, yoga – consult local adult education institute, women's centre, citizens' advice bureaux etc.

Hypnotherapy – consult the British Society of Hypnotherapists, 37 Orbain Road, London, SW6.

Relaxation/self-hypnosis tapes available from many sources (for example, health food shops and bookshops)

'New Age' music and awareness tapes can be obtained from New World Cassettes, PO Box 15, Twickenham, TW1 4SP (who also have a shop in Covent Garden)

In America, 'self-esteem' cassettes are available from:
Instar Communications
20 Sunnyside Avenue
Suite A-199
Mill Valley
CA 94941
USA
Tel: 800 544 7734

Marcia Germaine Hutchinson has also produced a set of seven 90-minute tapes entitled 'Transforming Body Image: learning to love the body you have'. A catalogue is available from:
Mind-Body Tapes
88 West Goulding Street
Sherborn
MA 01770
USA

Counselling

Send SAE to British Association for Counselling
37a Sheep Street
Rugby
CV21 3BX
Tel: 0788 78328

Co-counselling

Send SAE for directory to Co-counselling Phoenix
Change Strategies
5 Victoria Road
Sheffield
S10 2DJ

Eating Disorders Association
Sackville Place
44 Magdalen Street
Norwich
NR3 1JE
Tel: 0603 621414 9–4 pm, Mon–Fri, or 0494 21431 12–2 pm, Mon–Fri

Assertiveness training classes (countrywide, men and women)

Redwood Women's Training Association
Invergarry
Kitlings Lane
Walton-on-the-Hill
Stafford ST17 0LE
(send £1 for programme of classes)

Further reading

Transforming Body Image, Marcia Germaine Hutchinson (Freedom, California: Crossing Press, 1985)
The Big Beauty Book, Ann Harper and Glenn Lewis (New York: Holt, Rinehart and Winston, 1982)
Big and Beautiful, Ruthanne Olds (Washington DC: Acropolis Books, 1984)
Fat is a Feminist Issue, Susie Orbach (London: Arrow, 2nd edn 1988)
Fat is a Feminist Issue 2, Susie Orbach (London: Arrow, 1984)
The Mind Gymnasium, Denis Postle (London: Papermac, 1989)
Beyond Fear, Dorothy Rowe (London: Fontana, 1987)
Be Assertive, Beverley Hare (London: Macdonald Optima, 1988)

Self-Assertion for Women, Pamela E. Butler (New York: Harper & Row, 1982)

Dressing Thin, Dale Goday (1980)

Breaking all the Rules, Nancy Roberts (New York: Viking, 1985)

Awareness through Movement: Health Exercises for Personal Growth, M. Feldenkrais (New York: Harper and Row, 1977). Outlines the Feldenkrais method of awareness through movement

8

As We See It: Case Studies

This chapter is an 'open house': a forum for hopes and fears, troubles and triumphs, experiences and practical advice. All the people whose stories are told here have in some degree come to terms with their body size, but not without problems along the way. Perhaps you, like me, will recognize some of yourself in their feelings and experiences.

Annette

Annette is in her early 40s, and works as a sales training manager in London. She has a teenage family and is happily married to her second husband, Gary – otherwise known as retired wrestler 'Catweazle'. She is a contented size 28.

Life has not always been good for Annette. At sixteen, she weighed 63 kg (10 stone) and thought she was gross. Then she became pregnant. Desperate to hide the pregnancy, she put on weight deliberately and has never since been able to lose it. For years she was continually on and off diets, sometimes starving and sometimes eating for comfort. Her marriage was unhappy, she had little money and felt an utter failure. To quote Annette:

> When I was with my first husband, I didn't have much money and couldn't buy nice clothes. I felt I didn't deserve to anyway. Consequently I dressed badly. If I went out in the street I used to get called names by the children. I was mortified and terrified. I felt that I was just a blob, and that was how people saw me. People often think that you can't feel – that you cease to be a human being because you're fat.
>
> My first husband used to delight in humiliating me, and gave me a very, very poor self-image. He said that I was on Earth to see how far the human skin could stretch. Gradually, I began to believe that I had no right to exist at all.

Annette's life changed completely when she met Gary. Suddenly she realized that not everyone saw her in a negative, destructive way: 'My second husband is totally the opposite of my first. Being a wrestler, he thinks of big as being beautiful and normal. He hopes it doesn't harm my health, but he's quite happy about my size.'

Once in a loving, stable relationship, Annette began to learn to value herself as her husband clearly did. With greater self-confidence came a good job, and with the job came the money to buy attractive, stylish outfits which made the most of her figure. She is now complimented frequently on her appearance, and delights in wearing the luxurious, the unconventional and even the downright out-rageous. Gary has every confidence in her ability to create her own inimitable style: 'She could walk out in the street with a bowl on her head and get away with it,' he grins.

The ability to spend money on stylish and original clothes has become very important to Annette:

When I'm dressed well, I feel brilliant. If I'm not dressed well, I start feeling like a slob and some of the old doubts and insecurities slip back. Ken Smith has been an inspiration to me. When I discovered his designs, I realized that I could actually start wearing clothes that were *better* than most other people's. He may be a thin little man but I think he's wonderful! He produces stylish, quality clothes which last for years. I used to look like a ragbag, but not any more.

Annette sees clothing as a major problem for all large people, especially women: 'If you could wear the same clothes as smaller women, you wouldn't feel so different,' she points out. 'If only clothes manufacturers would wake up. There's a great mass of people out there, just waiting to part with their money.'

Work has also been a great source of confidence for Annette. Her weight has never been mentioned, and she enjoys an excellent working relationship with her colleagues and employers. She attributes some of her success to her strategy: 'I think that people see you the way you see yourself, so I tell everybody that I'm wonderful. I know that if I tell enough people they will end up believing it – and they do. If you put forward a positive image, people will accept it.'

All in all, Annette is contented with her life – though there are many areas in which she is striving for change: theatre seats, public transport, restaurants – all these are problems for large people, and she believes that large people must 'stand up and make a noise' in order to change society and its attitudes. As she herself says:

Fat women tend to stay quiet, accept what they are given and think they have no right to demand what everyone else has got. If they would only stand up and be counted. . . . It's possible to be big and happy, and I am. I'd prefer to be a bit smaller, but I don't think being thin is particularly desirable. Big can be beautiful if it's allowed to be.

Carmel and John

Carmel and John live near Hull, where Carmel is a staunch campaigner against fat oppression. Carmel, who is 30, used to work as a full-time welfare rights officer in a citizens' advice bureau. She has fluctuated between a size 12 and a size 24, but has now stabilized since giving up dieting. John describes himself as 'medium large'.

Carmel spent most of her adolescence and early adulthood on the dieting treadmill – sometimes losing weight but more often than not putting it all back on again (plus a bit more). At one point, she weighed 44 kg (7 stone) and was able to slip into a pair of size 10 jeans.

Her parents were a major influence on her decision to diet:

They were very critical of my size, and encouraged me to diet. I think that they were proudest of me when I was thin and therefore 'presentable'. They set great store by appearance and the clothes people wear – more, perhaps, than they should.

My mother put me on my first diet and, in effect, started my downward spiral into depression and misery. Until I left secondary school and was first made aware of my size, I liked myself. As soon as I began dieting and watching what I ate, I hated myself. I weighed myself every day and knew the calorie values of everything in the shops – so much so that I was a pain in the neck to be with!

My mother is a very attractive woman. She's also very intelligent, and I can understand her motives. She thought that I'd be happier and more able to enjoy my youth if I was 'normal' like the other girls. I care a great deal for her, and wish that she could accept me as I am. I believe that she needs to be able to accept herself too, because I feel that she too is under pressure to stay slim and dress well. She feels such guilt if she enjoys her food, or if she eats something high in calories and delicious – and that to me is a serious problem that she should resolve in order to enjoy life.

Now that she has ditched the diet sheets, Carmel feels she has a much better attitude to life:

> I have at last reached the conclusion that I like food. I enjoy eating and drinking and hate starving myself – and that's why I'm fat. My husband likes me as I am now, although he has known me when I was a slim size 12. In fact I think he prefers me now because I am a nicer person and am more easygoing if I am able to eat freely and have a good relationship with food.
>
> If I know that I am restricted in my food intake and can't have certain things, I suffer 'withdrawal symptoms' and become irritable. I'm cross if I'm hungry, so if I know I can eat normally and not feel guilty I'm a more likeable person to be with – and I like myself if I'm pleasant to be with.

John agrees that size is not a factor which he has ever taken into account in relationships:

> I have no preference for fat or thin women. But better a fat, intelligent, pleasant woman than a thin, unpleasant idiot. It's what's between the ears that counts, not the weight. I find some large women unattractive – I have no real hang-up about them, and I'm sceptical about 'mother-figure' theories.

Carmel believes that her self-confidence has been greatly increased through attending the Fat Women's Conference, and by reading Shelley Bovey's book, *Being Fat is not a Sin*. Both, she feels, have given her 'ammunition and strength to challenge oppression':

> The conference changed my life. The women who were there made me realize that I was a person with rights and that I was the equal of any thin woman. I learned an awful lot from that one day, and I want to share that with other women.

Another factor in her change of outlook is the assertiveness course which she attended in 1989: 'The group taught me that I don't have to take any old rubbish from anyone, and that I can say "enough is enough" whenever I choose.'

Media stereotypes infuriate Carmel, but she does have a heroine – actress Roseanne Barr: 'She has shown me – and probably thousands of other women – that talent is not exclusive to thin people, and that fat women have the right to be taken seriously, to be loved, and to be happy.'

As a 'medium large' man, John has also felt pressures on him to be thin – but has always found dieting extremely difficult. He is not against dieting, but says he would much rather be 'a fat nice guy than a thin jerk'. He is adamant that size need not be a barrier to forming good relationships:

> Be a good, kind, loving person and you will form relationships with the same sort of people. Being fat is not an insurmountable barrier to happiness. Only fools cannot see beyond a fake ideal of acceptable size. A person worth loving will love you whatever you look like if you can be a good person.
>
> Give love, and it will be returned ten times over. Think less about your own hangups and give love and affection to all you meet, and things will fall into place. It sounds trite, but it worked for me. We all have to find our own way through life, but love, openmindedness and affection are pretty good general rules.

For the future, Carmel and John plan to live life to the full, irrespective of their size. To quote Carmel:

> I can be happy as I am now, and I am not putting anything off until I am thin because I'll never be thin – and I'm not sure that I want to be. I believe in getting on with life now. Why wait until you are thin to do something you want to do now? Time passes so fast that, if you ever do become thin, it's too late to do whatever it is you wanted to do in the first place.

Danny

Danny (short for Danuta) is 40 years old and a size 24. She is married with two grown-up children, and usually does factory work. She lives in Lincolnshire.

As a young child, Danny sometimes went hungry, and she believes that this is one of the reasons why she ultimately became big:

> I had a fear of food running out for years afterwards, so I tended to eat 'extra today in case there isn't any tomorrow'. Also I frequently ate for comfort when depressed or under stress – a trait I have almost come to grips with, as I no longer bother with diets but have not gained any weight since March 1989.

144

Like Carmel, Danny feels her mother's attitude was a strong influence on her self-image as an adolescent:

> I spent my teenage years convinced I was a fat freak. 'Oh no! *You* can't wear full lace sleeves,' she would say, 'Not with *your* figure'; or 'I don't know how you can think of buying jeans', and so on. Recently I looked out some old photos and was quite shocked to discover that I was a fairly average sort of size 12–14, and not a balloon-woman after all.

Throughout her life, Danny has encountered negative reactions to her size – particularly, she says, from other women:

> They are worse than the men. A few have even been downright hostile – 'It's just disgusting, letting oneself go like that', or 'How can you expect a man to stay faithful if you look like that?'. About 50 per cent of women I meet hint at, or blatantly suggest, diets – often loudly and in front of other women. I used to get upset and feel guilty, but now I tend to reply 'Well, I notice you have a problem with your long nose/crooked teeth/out-of-condition hair, but I am not usually rude enough to go on about it in public.' A good conversation-stopper!

Apart from verbal insults, Danny is tired of coping with the host of practical problems that face large women in western society: clothes, job discrimination, media stereotypes, access and so on. She has particularly grim memories of trying to squeeze into fixed seating in burger bars like Wimpy and McDonalds. According to Danny:

> The main problems facing women are (a) brainwashing of themselves and their smaller sisters by advertising, fashion magazines, diet manufacturers, etc; (b) lack of confidence partly caused by above; (c) criticism by others who undermine said confidence; (d) ignorance of the facts about overweight, leading to self-criticism.

With the cards so definitively stacked against her, you might imagine that Danny was depressed. Not so! These days, Danny feels good about her body and intensely relieved to have escaped from the dieting treadmill:

> Since reading a book called *Overcoming Overeating*, I have

renounced all diets, forever. If I'm hungry I eat exactly what I want, so I no longer crave 'forbidden' things – there are *no* forbidden foods. My slim friends all predicted I'd 'balloon up', but much to their disgust I haven't put on a pound. And oh! The feeling of freedom! It's like losing a straightjacket.

Danny now realizes that she has achieved all her goals in life – without being thin – while many of the thin women she works with suffer all sorts of problems:

Working in a factory, I get to see large numbers of ordinary women and – as the work is undemanding mentally – a lot of talking is done, so I get to hear about their lives. I realized after a while that quite a lot of the ones I'd envied for their looks had bad marriages, or couldn't hold down relationships; their kids gave them no respect; some couldn't handle money; some were bored and always whining, but never doing anything about it. The list could be endless, but anyway, all these girls had their lives in a mess one way or another, and there was I – whose fat should equate with failure – doing OK, thank you. All I really wanted from life I've got: happy home life, kids I can relate to, good friends and enough to live on.

Looking at her life, Danny realized that she had unique talents and achievements – that she was by no means the 'fat failure' society would have her believe:

I discovered that I can do things that other people can't, like playing a musical instrument, doing handicrafts, and writing poems and songs. I found out that the people I looked upon as slim supergirls were actually *envying* me!

Danny enjoys life to the full, and – although she has never seen herself as 'sporty' – she keeps fit and supple with plenty of walking and swimming. She even takes part in the occasional football match or sponsored event 'if it's for charity'.

Her advice to other large people is:

Really think about other people's lives. Take your friend who's fat, too. Do you think she's awful, lazy, stupid and ugly? Probably not. So why think you are? Think about the thin girl you know. Is her life perfect? Has she no faults, no problems? Think of your achievements: all the things you've succeeded in. You did it all as a fat person. You didn't need slimness to do any of it.

This incident might serve to illustrate the irony of it all. There's a woman where I work – she's size 8–10, has a nice face, decent personality. Lots of us envied her looks and a lot of the women there think you need looks to keep a man interested.

Well, last week she bought a very sexy new dress – strappy top, with the skirt made of long 'petals' that separate as you move. She was showing her friends at tea break, and I could hear remarks like 'Wish I had the figure to wear that'. Then a couple of the men went by, and I heard one say to the other, 'Gawd – I've seen more meat on a chicken bone!'. The others laughed. Can't win, can you?

Anita

Anita is 56, and she is 1.7 m (5'8½"–9") tall and a size 24. She is a JP, trained silversmith and jeweller, and also works part-time in an Oxfam shop. Her husband is an academic, and she has four children aged 26 to 33. She lives in Sheffield.

Anita was always a tall, robust girl, but didn't have a 'weight problem' until she contracted polio at the age of 16:

> It was lying on my back for months on end, and not walking for two years, that did it. . . . At that time, they 'built you up' in hospital, so I found I was given food about every two or three hours – and consequently, I got used to feeling full. . . . My mother had always wanted a small 'fairy daughter', and was ashamed of my fat, which of course contributed to my great unhappiness. I think she was more or less anorexic herself, and considered it a sin to have butter as well as jam on your bread.

As a tall woman as well as a large one, Anita feels she has a double problem. Rather than making her shy and reticent, her size tends to make her appear rather aggressive: 'Because I'm tall and big all over, I find it's likely to make me seem overbearing.'

As she suffers from high blood pressure, Anita and her general practitioner believe that she would feel healthier if she lost weight. Unfortunately, a series of unsuccessful diets in the past have made her a victim of the 'yo-yo syndrome' – losing weight and then putting it all back on again – which can be even more dangerous than remaining at a constantly high weight.

For years, Anita tried different diets, and finally ended up at Weight Watchers: 'I lost 33 kg (4½ stone) with them, and I thought I'd never put it back on. I was wrong. My feeling is that Weight Watchers is dangerous, because it makes you obsessed with food. I was forever weighing and thinking about food. If I hadn't got food I was wondering what I could have when I had it – and this really did become an obsession. So I said "never again", and put the 33 kg (4½ stone) back on.'

Anita's solution to her problem came in the form of a collection of books on high-fibre diets which arrived at the Oxfam shop one day. In desperation she bought them, and found that a programme of sensible, high-fibre eating was a real help to her. Over a period of three months she has lost about 11 kg (2 stone) without consciously dieting; so she is hoping that she has found a healthy eating plan that she can stick to for the rest of her life without the terrible sense of deprivation which comes from 'crash' diets.

Whether or not she ever becomes thinner, Anita has no intention of letting her size stop her from leading an active life. At an age when many ladies are thinking about retirement, Anita is setting out to do all the things she has always wanted to do:

> I feel more strongly now than ever before, because two of my great friends – both in their 40s – recently died of cancer, and I feel that they didn't lead their lives to the full. I'm absolutely determined to do that. There's simply nothing I don't do. I've just come back from a walking holiday with my husband in Switzerland. Every day we did 20–24 km (12–15 miles) up and down hills in the heat. I've been hitchhiking with my son for five blissful weeks in Nepal. The year after that, he said 'Meet me in Turkey in 24 hours'. Off I went, and hitchhiked round Turkey with him.
>
> I bike, walk and do a lot of swimming. I swim in the University pool and it's never worried me. We all have showers together, but I've never quite managed to take off my swimsuit: I've decided this is quite ridiculous and I'm going to try and cure it.

According to Anita, the important thing is to remember that you only have one life, and it's foolish to spoil it by running yourself down:

> It's very easy to wallow in your fatness and think all your problems are because you're fat. I know people who think all their problems are because they're Jewish, or because they didn't go to public school, or because they can't stop blushing. You can have many

complexes about being fat, because it's a useful hook to hang them on. I don't think it has to be so. I think you can make anything a disability and an excuse for not living life to the full. Fat is just one of them, and it's dangerous to rest everything on it.

Anita's advice to other large people is:

Come on: get out there and live. You only live once, so enjoy it. I find life extremely exciting, and it's getting better and better. In some ways, being older helps because you seem to forget worrying about things and just get on with living. It's all a question of how you see yourself. Why should you adapt to others? Why should they adapt to you? Your life is yours. I can live with someone's smoking, or with their big ears or crooked nose. If they can't live with my being fat, bad luck to them.

Index